100 Questions & Answers About Menopause

Ivy M. Alexander, PhD, C-ANP
Yale University School of Nursing

Karla A. Knight, RN, MSN
Nursing Spectrum

JONES AND BARTLETT PUBLISHERS
Sudbury, Massachusetts
BOSTON   TORONTO   LONDON   SINGAPORE

World Headquarters

Jones and Bartlett
Publishers
40 Tall Pine Drive
Sudbury, MA 01776
info@jbpub.com
www.jbpub.com

Jones and Bartlett
Publishers Canada
2406 Nikanna Road
Mississauga, ON L5C 2W6
CANADA

Jones and Bartlett
Publishers International
Barb House, Barb Mews
London W6 7PA
UK

Library of Congress Cataloging-in-Publication Data
Alexander, Ivy M.
    100 questions & answers about menopause / Ivy M. Alexander, Karla A. Knight.
        p. cm.
    Includes index.
    ISBN 0-7637-2729-6 (pbk.)
    1. Menopause—Popular works. 2. Menopause—Miscellanea. I. Title: One hundred questions and answers about menopause. II. Knight, Karla A. III. Title.
    RG186.A43 2005
    618.1'75—dc22

                                        2004029535

Production Credits
Chief Executive Officer: Clayton Jones
Chief Operating Officer: Don W. Jones, Jr.
President, Higher Education and Professional Publishing: Robert W. Holland, Jr.
V.P., Sales and Marketing: William J. Kane
V.P., Design and Production: Anne Spencer
V.P., Manufacturing and Inventory Control: Therese Bräuer
Executive Publisher: Christopher Davis
Production Director: Amy Rose
Special Projects Editor: Elizabeth Platt
Editorial Assistant: Kathy Richardson
Marketing Manager: Matthew Payne
Composition: Northeast Compositors
Cover Design: Colleen Halloran
Cover Image: © Ryan McVay/Photodisc/Getty Images
Printing and Binding: Malloy, Inc.
Cover Printing: Malloy, Inc.

Printed in the United States of America
09 08 07 06 05   10 9 8 7 6 5 4 3 2 1

Contents

Part 1: An Overview of Menopause   1

Questions 1–14 describe the physiology and hormonal changes associated with menopause, including:

- What is menopause?
- How long can I expect to menstruate? Can I predict when I'll have my final menstrual period?
- What other circumstances can cause menopause?
- What is a hysterectomy, and how does it affect menopause?

Part 2: Experiencing the Symptoms of Menopause   29

Questions 15–33 address hot flashes, irregular menstrual periods, mood changes, inability to sleep, decreased sexual drive, weight gain, and other symptoms related to menopause, including:

- What kind of symptoms can I expect to experience as I transition into menopause?
- What is a hot flash?
- What causes me to be so irritable and cry so easily?
- Why do I seem to forget things more easily?
- Why can't I get a good night's sleep?

Part 3: Evaluating Symptoms: Is It Menopause?   63

Questions 34–53 address the importance of having certain symptoms and other midlife health risks evaluated by your healthcare provider, including:

- Are there health problems that I should be screened for as I approach menopause and after?
- What is osteoporosis? I've heard that I'm at greater risk for it during menopause. Is that true? Why am I more at risk for osteoporosis during postmenopause?
- How do I know if I'm depressed?
- Am I more likely to get breast, endometrial, ovarian, or cervical cancer after menopause?

Every woman experiences menopause in a different way. Some women glide through the menopausal transition and never have any symptoms at all. However, many women have symptoms that can substantially interfere with their quality of life. There are women who don't sleep well or wake up soaked with perspiration. There are women who complain of being forgetful and are concerned that their memory will fail them forever. Many women have vaginal symptoms that can make sex painful or can even make sitting uncomfortable. In addition, other changes in the urogenital tract can increase urinary infections and incontinence.

There are a few things that every woman with a uterus will experience. A change in menstrual patterns is one of those common experiences. These changes may include changes in the frequency of menstrual periods and often the amount of bleeding. Ultimately, periods will stop altogether. Although many of the symptoms of menopause start years before a woman's final period, a woman is not truly menopausal until she hasn't had a period for one year.

Some women view the loss of their periods and fertility with great relief. For these women, freedom from pregnancy as well as the freedom from periods are welcomed. Other women view these changes as a loss of their youth or regret not being able to become pregnant again (or ever). The physical and emotional changes surrounding menopause cannot be predicted for any woman. Every woman is different.

There is one thing that all women entering menopause have— questions and more questions. This book answers 100 of the most common questions that women have about menopause, including some questions they may not have thought of but should consider. Written by a nurse practitioner and a nurse, this book gives practical answers and helpful tips on staying healthy and happy through this important physical and sometimes emotional transition. It helps women to understand what to expect and what is normal during this time. More importantly, it addresses health issues that are far more common in women after menopause, such as vaginal dryness, urinary incontinence, heart palpitations, dry eyes, and joint and muscle aches. It also addresses more serious problems such as osteoporosis, heart disease, obesity, and other health problems that can often be prevented with the right plan of action.

The choices about what to do about menopausal symptoms can be daunting. This book provides straight answers about choices that a woman might be considering and what those benefits and risks might be for her. The information provided here goes well beyond the headlines about hormone therapy and gives an accurate perspective about what the studies about hormones have shown to date. In addition, alternatives to hormones are also provided so every choice can be considered.

So whether it is finding out what is normal during the menopause transition, finding out how to relieve symptoms, or learning how to stay healthy in the second half of life, this well organized, easy-to-read book will answer many of a woman's questions.

Use this book to have your questions answered, and have a happy and healthful menopause.

Susan Wysocki, RNC, NP
President and CEO
National Association of Nurse Practitioners in Women's Health

Like many readers, I, too, sat at the breakfast table in the summer of 2002 and listened to the confusing morass of media advising me that the Women's Health Initiative (WHI) had been shut down. Like many of you, that was all I heard at first gulp. This large study was being stopped prematurely due to unacceptable side effects, particularly related to breast cancer. Unlike many of you, I am a women's health nurse practitioner. Hormone therapy (HT) had been the standard of care for the 20 years that I had been practicing. What was going to become of all of my menopausal patients, my friends, and of course, self-centeredly, me?

HT was then and is now part of the many tools available for handling symptoms and some of the diseases that occur in women as they age. We know now that there is no "magic bullet" to maintaining our health and maximizing our independence. As a women's health specialist, I had an advantage of being familiar with many of the previous studies, and had a basis for comparing the data and the very confusing statistical analyses. If I was troubled and at times confused, I can only imagine the concerns among my patients and my friends. I know from experience that many women stopped their HT "cold turkey" that morning. Others were concerned that this was a promulgation of women as underdogs, and that unscrupulous drug companies were manipulating us.

Ivy Alexander and Karla Knight have tackled the huge topic of menopause since the WHI and produced this very easy-to-read, informative book. While not intended to replace any dialogue with your healthcare provider, this book can provide the platform for very spirited and informed discussions. This book focuses on the answers to the many questions, ranging from simple to difficult, about HT, aging, and life after your ovaries cease to produce estrogen. It addresses the "new paradigm" of using HT to its best bene-fits. The authors provide insightful options that are lifestyle man-agement changes rather than pharmaceutical. There is information about alternative and complementary therapies as well. It is written in a format that does not require your diligence in reading it cover to cover, rather allowing the reader to use the question-and-answer format to direct your reading to your specific concerns. You can refer to the symptom table and be directed to particular portions of the book.

I hope this book finds its way to the bookshelves of the many women who are embracing the many decades of their lives beyond their ability to reproduce and menstruate. It will be an asset to those women, as well as to those women who are approaching the next phase more cautiously and with some trepidation. The answers to your questions are all found here. I hope you enjoy this book, and find confidence and wisdom in the information that is provided.

Kay Hood, WHNP, PhD
Ponte Vedra Beach, Florida

Why write a book about menopause? Because menopause affects every woman in some way or another—yes, you might be saying, as you fan yourself during a hot flash. But menopause is bigger than just symptoms. It is a transition in life that many women embrace. It is often a time for reflection and reevaluation, and can serve as a catalyst for changing lifestyles and improving health.

More women are entering menopause every day, and the amount of time that women live beyond menopause is increasing. Women experience not only menopausal symptoms at midlife, but their health risks change. Helping women effectively manage menopause symptoms and maintain their health is increasingly important. This is not easy to accomplish. Deciding on the best approach has become more complex with new research information and recent controversies. There has also been a trend in the United States toward using complementary and alternative therapies, but little research is available to educate us about the effectiveness and safety of some of these treatments. The more we learn about possible methods for managing menopausal symptoms and midlife health risks, the more complicated management selection becomes.

I first developed an interest in menopause because of my patients. As the population of women I care for ages, and they experience menopausal symptoms and develop problems that are more commonly seen in midlife (such as osteoporosis, heart disease, and diabetes), I have become increasingly interested in prevention and management of menopause and midlife health risks.

Through my research and from my patients, I have learned that menopause is a mystery to most women. Symptoms are unpredictable, distressing, and confusing. You never know when hot flashes might occur, and you don't have any idea how long they will last. Menopause is rarely discussed in the open. Most women learn about menopause by talking with friends, mothers, or aunts, or by seeking information on their own. I am struck by the amount of misinformation that is easily accessible, as well as the lack of accurate and balanced information. So I jumped at the opportunity to write this book.

It is our goal to provide you with understandable and truthful information about menopause, to provide a realistic picture that fairly portrays both the challenges and rewards, and to share information that you can use to make informed decisions about your own health. We want to provide you with balanced, accurate information about possible symptom-management strategies, including lifestyle changes, hormone therapy, and complementary and alternative treatments. Because of this we have included a bibliography listing many of the references and resources that we used to write this book. Research information about specific strategies is an important part of understanding how well a specific strategy might work. This information is intended to help you make informed decisions about treatment options, and we hope that you will read about future research as more information becomes available. We recognize that this book is one of many sources of information about menopause. We encourage you to use it in addition to these other sources, talk with friends and family members, and consider carefully the many options that are available to you. And we hope you will use the information presented here in discussions with your clinicians.

I truly enjoyed the process of writing this book. Karla and I had telephone conferences every week. During these discussions we learned more about menopause and about each other—and the process of writing as a team! It has been a fun, exhausting, and exhilarating project.

Many people assisted us in making this book a reality. I owe special appreciation to the women who have shared their stories with me. Some of their stories are included in this book, using pseudonyms to protect their confidentiality. I am grateful to Linda Bell, Registered Dietician; Dave Brzozowski and Mark Theriault, Clinical Pharmacists; and several other colleagues and friends who shared their expertise. Thanks also to Chris Davis, Kathy Richardson, and Elizabeth Platt at Jones and Bartlett Publishers, Inc., who have provided sage advice and guidance.

I would never have completed this book without the encouragement of my many colleagues and friends. Last, but definitely not least, I want to thank my family—for their encouragement, support, and, most of all, understanding throughout this process.

—Ivy M. Alexander

When I first started thinking about writing this book, my husband and I were watching a TV sitcom in which a frenzied, supposedly menopausal housekeeper could not care for the children one day because she was very irritable and eating everything in sight. The children were pleading not to be left alone with her. My husband said, "That's not a very good advertisement for menopause!"

But in some ways, women have been sold a bill of goods. They expect that they are going to have terrible hot flashes, drenching sweats, and brittle bones. They expect that they'll never want sex again. They are going to become wrinkled and die from heart disease. Mood swings will make their lives miserable. Menopause's reputation is hardly glamorous. And yet some women sail through it, either wondering what the fuss is all about, or making the women who experience lots of symptoms feel worse. In reality, menopause is an individual experience for everyone. One day you'll think you'll never be able to cope; the next, you're on top of the world.

This book may not provide the answers to all of your questions about menopause or your health at midlife. Many times you will be able to use the suggestions in the book to help yourself. Other times, however, it will be necessary and important to call your clinician. Because this book is not a substitute for health care or for the management of menopause, you will note that we refer often to seeing your clinician. This is not a cop-out; this is good practice. It is important for you to feel comfortable discussing symptoms and treatments with your clinician.

My co-author Ivy and I met when I was writing an article about women's health for *Nursing Spectrum.* She spoke eloquently about the issues facing women, particularly at midlife. So when Kathy Richardson, my friend and neighbor of 21 years, asked me to consider writing a book on menopause, I knew instantly that Ivy would make a great co-author. Thank you, Ivy, for agreeing to write this book with me. I will miss our weekly conversations about menopause and life in general.

I never imagined when Kathy and I went for one of our evening walks, talking about all the things that girlfriends talk about, that she would ask me to write a book about menopause. Thanks, Kathy, for your guidance and support all along the book-writing journey. You have always known how important it is to write something that all women could understand and relate to.

My family, immediate and extended, has provided support in all sorts of ways, particularly when my own perimenopausal symptoms kicked in. Thank you, Erin, for making me laugh at my "temperature deregulations" while I insisted I wasn't having hot flashes. Kyle, thanks for sharing the computer this past summer while you were also writing a book. Thanks, Kelsey, for asking your grandmother about my quick-to-tears temperament. Her suggestion that I might need some estrogen gave me a chance to talk to you about menopause! Thanks, Tom, for always being the understanding and wonderful husband that you are.

Acknowledgments of friends and colleagues by name would be lengthy. But you know who you are and how much I appreciate your support. Whether by phone, e-mail, or in person, you've all been great, and in your own ways, have contributed so much to this book.

—Karla A. Knight

We dedicate this book to you, the woman experiencing menopause, and your family—we hope you find it informative and helpful. We also dedicate this book to the many women who were willing to share their stories about menopause and who taught us what is important, especially to those who have provided comments that are included in these pages.

PART ONE

An Overview
of Menopause

What is menopause?

How long can I expect to menstruate? Can I predict
when I'll have my final menstrual period?

What other circumstances can cause menopause?

What is a hysterectomy, and how does it affect
menopause?

More . . .

1. What is menopause?

Menopause is medically defined as the specific point in time following 12 consecutive months without a **menstrual period**. However, most women describe themselves as "in menopause" when they start to experience symptoms of the menopausal transition such as **irregular periods**, **hot flashes**, and mood changes.

Natural menopause happens to every woman who lives long enough, and for whom menopause is not caused by surgery or by other means, such as chemotherapy.

Menopause may be a time of body changes, mood swings, and thoughts of aging, but it can also be a time of reflection, a time of taking stock of one's life. Menopause has also been described as the transition from the reproductive to the nonreproductive phase of a woman's life.

Menopause is often called "the change," "change of life," or "the Big M." No matter what you call it, the word "menopause" conjures up many reactions and emotions among those who experience it. These responses often vary among the women who are living through menopause, as well as among their partners and family members. The clinical definition of menopause does not begin to describe the **physiologic** changes, the symptoms, or the emotional responses that accompany it.

Menopause

specific point in time occurring after 12 consecutive months without a menstrual period that does not have another identifiable cause such as illness or medication.

Menstrual period

blood flow that occurs approximately every 28 to 30 days in a reproductive-aged woman when the top layer of the lining of the internal uterus wall sheds.

Irregular periods

period that is shorter, longer, lighter, or heavier-than-usual period.

Hot flashes

sensations of heat that often begin at the head and spread over the entire body; accompanies perimenopause and postmenopause for many women.

Physiologic

pertaining to body function.

Menopause, although technically a point in time, is a natural life transition. The way you experience menopause is very individual, but you don't have to go through it alone. In fact, if you have reached menopause—that point where you have not had a period for 12 consecutive months—you were joined by about 5,000 other women today!

Menopause, although technically a point in time, is a natural life transition.

Trina's comment:

Menopause. Well…you could read ten articles on it and end up with ten different descriptions. For me, menopause means lots of symptoms: hot flashes, sweats, trouble sleeping, moodiness, crying for no reason. I get so exhausted from not sleeping that I feel lucky getting to work safely some days. And sex, forget it. Menopause means 'men-o-pause'—I'm just not interested. When it first started I didn't know what was going on. It's like a taboo; the generation before us never discussed it. I didn't even know what was wrong with me. I thought I had some terrible disease. But no, it's just menopause, lucky me—ha! Some days I feel like it has taken over my life—I am too tired to go out, I'm not interested in sex, and sometimes I get really down about the whole thing. But then I try to remember that it is just a natural part of life, another thing I have to go through, and I try not to let it get the best of me.

2. What are perimenopause and postmenopause?

The time period before menopause during which symptoms of hormonal changes occur is called **perimenopause**. While some women may experience nothing more than irregular periods in the years leading up to their **final menstrual period (FMP)**, many

Perimenopause
time period before and up to menopause including the 12 months of no menses when symptoms of hormonal changes occur; can last up to 8 to 10 years.

Final menstrual period (FMP)
the last menstrual period before menopause. Like menopause, the FMP can only be identified in hindsight.

Ovulation

release of an egg (ovum) from the ovary stimulated by luteinizing hormone; usually occurs approximately 14 days before the first day of the menstrual period.

women experience a variety of symptoms during perimenopause. Although perimenopause is a time when **ovulation** occurs irregularly, it is still possible to get pregnant during this time.

The symptoms preceding the FMP can last from 2 to 8 years. See Table 1 for a list of symptoms commonly

Table 1   Symptoms Associated with Perimenopause and Postmenopause

Acne	Breast Pain	Creeping Sensation on Skin
Decreased Sex Drive	Depression	Dizziness
Dry Eyes	Dry/Thinning Hair	Fatigue
Forgetfulness	Headache	Hair Growth on Face
Hot Flashes/Flushes	Irregular Heart Beat	Irritability/Mood Disturbances
Irregular Menses/ Bleeding	Joint Pain	Muscle Aches
Muscle Weakness	Nervousness/Anxiety	Night Sweats
Nighttime Urination	Numbness	Odor
Painful Intercourse	Painful Urination	Poor Concentration
Recurrent Bladder Infections	Recurrent Vaginal Infections	Sleep Disturbances/ Insomnia
Skin Dryness	Stress Urinary Incontinence*	Tingling/Prickling Sensations
Urinary Frequency	Urinary Urgency	Vaginal Dryness
Vaginal/Vulvar Burning	Vaginal/Vulvar Irritation	Vaginal/Vulvar Itching

*Data are inconclusive.

associated with perimenopause, the **menopause transition**, and **postmenopause**.

It is difficult to predict how long perimenopause will last, but if you approach 50 without any symptoms, you are more likely to have a shorter perimenopause. The most prominent symptom of perimenopause is menstrual irregularities—meaning that menstrual periods can become heavier, longer, shorter, or lighter without any particular frequency or predictability.

Women are considered postmenopausal once menstrual periods have stopped for 12 consecutive months. That doesn't mean that symptoms also stop. Most women report having hot flashes for up to 7 years after their FMP, and a few women will experience symptoms longer. See Figure 1, which shows a timeline of typical ages for experiencing the first menstrual period, perimenopause symptoms, menopause, and postmenopause.

Some women go through perimenopause without any symptoms, so it is possible to get past menopause and wonder what all the fuss was about.

Menopause transition
the time period before and up to the final menstrual period when hormonal changes occur.

Postmenopause
the time period following menopause.

An Overview of Menopause

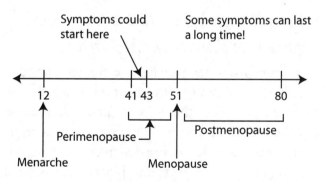

*Ages are approximate and based on averages and average life expectancy of 80.

Figure 1   A typical lifetime of menstrual changes and symptoms.*

3. What is estrogen?

Estrogen is known as the female sex hormone, although one form of estrogen is also found in men. There are three types of estrogen. **Estrone** (E1) is the main estrogen of the postmenopausal phase, and is also present in small amounts in men and children. **Estradiol** (E2) is the main estrogen during a woman's reproductive years, and is the strongest form of estrogen produced in the body. **Estriol** (E3) is the main estrogen of pregnancy and is secreted by the placenta. E1 and E3 are weak estrogens in comparison to E2.

Estrogen is responsible for the development of sex changes in girls, and for some of the changes in the vagina and **endometrial lining**. Rising levels of estrogen secreted by the ovaries precedes ovulation in a normal menstrual cycle.

Manufactured forms of estradiol are used in **estrogen therapy (ET)** and **estrogen progestin therapy (EPT)** for the treatment of perimenopausal and postmenopausal symptoms (see Part 5).

4. Why is it important to know about estrogen's role during menopause?

Estrogen receptors (sites where estrogen connects with body cells and through this connection affects cell function) are located in the body in such places as the parts of the brain that control thinking and heat regulation, the eyes, heart, lungs, breasts, liver, colon, reproductive organs, urinary system, blood vessels, and

Estrogen

a female sex hormone also found in men in small amounts. It is primarily secreted by the ovary in response to follicle stimulating hormone (FSH).

Estrone

the main estrogen of the postmenopausal phase, and is also present in small amounts in men and children. Also called E1.

Estradiol

the most potent of the naturally occurring estrogens in the human body and the main estrogen of the reproductive years. Also called E2.

Estriol

estriol (E3) is the main estrogen of pregnancy and is secreted by the placenta. It is also present in women who are not pregnant as a byproduct of E1 and E2.

Endometrial lining

the lining of the uterus that is shed during menstruation.

bone. There may be other receptor sites yet to be discovered. See Figure 2 for the body locations of receptor sites. There is growing evidence that estrogens have an important effect on these sites. The low levels of estrogen during postmenopause can be responsible for bone loss, urinary **incontinence**, decreased elasticity of skin and blood vessels, as well as the more familiar symptoms of hot flashes, night sweats, and vaginal dryness.

Estrogen levels are erratic during perimenopause and decreased following menopause. Women do continue to make low levels of estradiol and estrone during postmenopause, but not enough to stop the symptoms of menopause. Symptoms tend to increase during the first year after menopause because the greatest decline in estrogen production occurs around this time.

5. What is progesterone?

Progesterone is a sex hormone, and is responsible for the changes in the uterus especially during the last two weeks of the menstrual cycle when the uterine lining is prepared for a fertilized egg. If an egg does become fertilized, more progesterone is secreted to protect the pregnancy. An easy way to remember progesterone's role is that progesterone *pro*tects *gest*ation and it is a *ster*oid horm*one*. If an egg does not get fertilized, progesterone levels drop and **menstruation** usually begins. Like estrogen, progesterone is secreted by the ovaries and also has many receptors around the body. For progesterone, these receptors include the hypothalamus, pituitary gland, heart, lungs, breasts, pancreas,

Estrogen therapy (ET)
estrogen-containing products used in the treatment of perimenopausal and menopausal symptoms.

Estrogen progestin therapy (EPT)
estrogen- and progestin-containing products used in combination for the treatment of menopausal symptoms.

Estrogen receptors
sites in the human body where estrogen binds and affects cell functions.

Incontinence
inability to hold urine.

Progesterone
a female sex hormone that is responsible for the changes in the uterus, especially during the part of the menstrual cycle that is preparing the uterine lining for a fertilized egg, and helps to sustain pregnancy. It is also the female hormone that protects the endometrial lining of the uterus from thickening too much in response to estrogen.

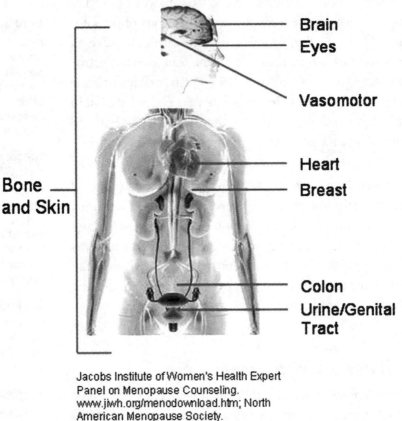

Brain

Eyes

Vasomotor

Heart

Breast

Bone and Skin

Colon

Urine/Genital Tract

Jacobs Institute of Women's Health Expert
Panel on Menopause Counseling.
www.jiwh.org/menodownload.htm; North
American Menopause Society.
www.menopause.org/edumaterials/guidebook
/mgtoc.html.

Figure 2   Estrogen receptors. (Reprinted with permission from Warner Chilcott, Inc.)

reproductive organs, blood vessels, bone, and the brain.
See Figure 3 for **progesterone receptor sites**.
Although fluctuations in progesterone levels are not as
clearly linked to perimenopause and menopausal
symptoms, it does play a role.

Manufactured progesterones, usually called **progestogens** or **progestins**, are used together with estrogen for treating symptoms of menopause (estrogen progestin therapy, EPT). In this book, we refer to progesterone as either the naturally occurring hormone in the body, or **bio-identical** manufactured hormones. Progestins are either bio-identical or synthetic manufactured progesterone hormones.

The main role of progesterone or progestin is to prevent overgrowth of the uterine lining (**endometrium**), which can increase the risk for **endometrial cancer**. If women take estrogen and still have a uterus, they must also take progesterone or a progestin. Progesterone cream applied **topically** (to the skin) does not have sufficient absorption to prevent the thickening of the uterine lining caused by taking estrogen. Thickening of the lining without a **withdrawal bleed** (a period) can cause **endometrial hyperplasia** and may lead to endometrial cancer.

6. What happens to hormones during a normal menstrual cycle?

In order to understand the effects of hormones during menopause, it is important to understand how hormones work during a normal menstrual cycle.

The menstrual cycle is regulated by both **positive and negative feedback systems**—meaning that certain hormones are released in response to either high or low levels of another hormone—in a loop called the

Menstruation

the process of discharging the blood and endometrial debris during the menstrual period.

Progesterone receptor sites

sites in the human body where progesterone binds and affects cell functions.

Progestogens

refers to either progesterone made in the body or to progestins manufactured for the purposes of hormone therapy.

Progestins

any manufactured progesterone; can be used to prevent overgrowth of the uterine lining to prevent the risk for endometrial cancer, stabilize the uterine lining during irregular bleeding, help manage menopause symptoms, and to sustain pregnancy.

An Overview of Menopause

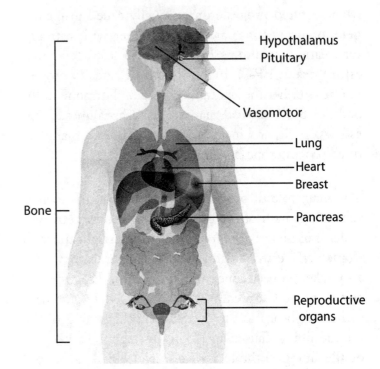

Figure 3   **Progesterone receptors. (Adapted from *The Color Atlas of Human Anatomy*, 1980. Reprinted with permission from Warner Chilcott, Inc.)**

Bio-identical hormones

hormones manufactured in a laboratory that have the exact same chemical makeup as the hormones made in the body. Sometimes called "natural" hormones.

Endometrium

the inner layer of the uterus. The lining of the endometrium is shed during menstruation.

Endometrial cancer

cancer of the lining of the uterus.

HPO axis (hypothalamus-pituitary-ovarian axis). The HPO axis is important to our understanding of menopause because disruptions in the axis are what eventually cause hormonal changes that are linked to the symptoms during perimenopause. See Figure 4.

At both the beginning and end of the average 28-day menstrual cycle, low levels of estrogen and progesterone prompt **gonadotropin-releasing hormone (GnRH)** to be secreted by the hypothalamus in the brain, which in turn causes **follicle-stimulating hormone (FSH)** to be released by the **anterior pituitary gland**, also in the brain. FSH stimulates a group of

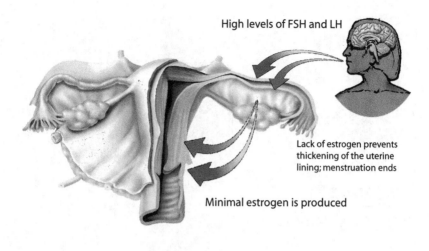

High levels of FSH and LH

Lack of estrogen prevents thickening of the uterine lining; menstruation ends

Minimal estrogen is produced

North American Menopause Society.
www.menopause.org/edumaterials/guidebook/mgtoc.html

Figure 4   Hypothalamus–pituitary–ovarian (HPO) axis approaching menopause. (Reprinted with permission from Warner Chilcott, Inc.)

follicles in the ovary to start producing **androgen,** and converting androgen to estrogen. Levels of FSH and estrogen continue to rise, forcing the follicles to grow. (This occurs during the first half of the menstrual cycle, the follicular phase.)

At about day 7 of the cycle, the largest follicle (the dominant follicle) takes over. Once estrogen gets to a high enough level, a "surge" or burst of LH (**luteinizing hormone**) from the anterior pituitary gland is released. The high estrogen together with the LH surge causes the dominant follicle to expel an egg (ovulation), which occurs 24 to 36 hours after the LH surge. The egg then makes the journey from the ovary to the **fallopian tube**.

Topically
applied to the skin.

Withdrawal bleeding

bleeding from the vagina that occurs after stopping progestin. This bleeding allows the lining of the uterus to shed.

Endometrial hyperplasia

abnormal thickening or overgrowth of the lining of the uterus. This may lead to cancer.

An Overview of Menopause

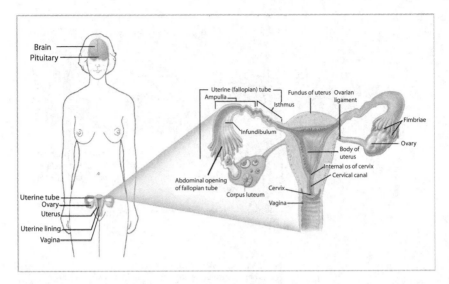

Figure 5 Female reproductive anatomy. (Adapted from Netter, *The Netter Collection of Medical Illustrations* 1997, and Williams et al., *Gray's Anatomy* 1995; reprinted with permission from Warner Chilcott, Inc.)

Positive and negative feedback systems

certain hormones or substances are released in response to either high or low levels of another hormone or substance.

HPO axis (hypothalamus-pituitary-ovarian axis)

the feedback system that regulates levels of estrogen, progesterone, follicle-stimulating hormone (FSH), gonadotropin-releasing hormone (GnRH), and luteinizing hormone.

After ovulation, the dominant follicle continues to make estrogen and progesterone. It is now called the **corpus luteum** because of its yellowish color caused by **lutein**. See Figure 5 for the anatomy. The corpus luteum will start to shrink about 10 or 11 days after ovulation, provided there is no fertilization of the egg. Estrogen and progesterone levels will also decline. The low levels of progesterone, and to a lesser degree estrogen, cause the uterine lining to shed. Menstruation occurs over the first 5 or so days of the cycle. See Figure 6 showing the normal hormone levels in a menstrual cycle.

If the egg is fertilized by sperm, a pregnancy occurs and the corpus luteum keeps on producing estrogen and progesterone. These sustained levels of estrogen

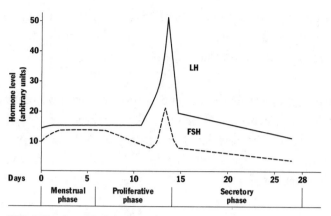

(A) Fluctuation of gonadotropin levels

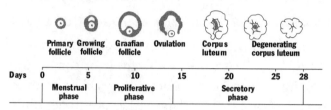

(B) Ovarian cycle

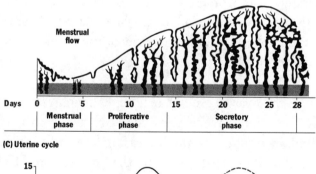

(C) Uterine cycle

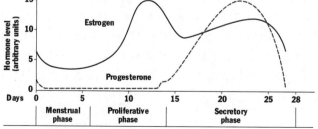

(D) Fluctuation of ovarian hormone levels

Figure 6   Hormone levels in the female menstrual cycle.

Gonadotropin-releasing hormone (GnRH)

a hormone that is released from the hypothalamus to stimulate production of luteinizing hormone (LH) and follicle stimulating hormone (FSH).

Follicle stimulating-hormone (FSH)

a hormone released from the anterior pituitary gland to stimulate the growth of follicles in the ovary. Estrogen levels also rise in response to FSH.

Anterior pituitary gland

the part of the pituitary gland, which is situated at the base of the brain, that releases follicle-stimulating hormone (FSH) and luteinizing hormone (LH) as part of the menstrual cycle.

Follicles

a sac of immature "eggs" in the ovary stimulated to grow by the follicle-stimulating hormone (FSH) and estrogen. When estrogen levels get high enough, luteinizing hormone (LH) is released too so that the dominant follicle expels a mature egg from the ovary.

and progesterone prevent GnRH and FSH from being released, and prevent the endometrial lining from shedding (no menstruation).

If the egg is not fertilized, the corpus luteum no longer produces hormones. Through the negative feedback mechanism, the low levels of estrogen tell the hypothalamus to start secreting GnRH again. And the cycle starts over.

7. What happens to the hormones of the menstrual cycle leading up to menopause?

The normal positive and negative feedback systems of the HPO axis don't work as effectively or consistently leading up to menopause. The ovaries' ability to make estrogen and progesterone diminishes over time, which also means that a normal menstrual cycle cannot be maintained. As women age, the follicles in the ovary are simply unable to produce the same levels of estrogen and progesterone as they did during peak reproductive years.

Because the ovaries are not making as much estrogen, GnRH continues to be released. FSH also continues to climb in response to the increasing levels of GnRH. Some clinicians used to think that measuring FSH was a good way to diagnose menopause. In reality, FSH levels may be elevated one day and normal the next during the perimenopause, so this is no longer considered a reliable way to identify menopause. (See Question 51 regarding FSH testing.)

"Hormonal chaos" is a term that describes the perimenopause including the 12 months or more that precede the actual point of menopause. At any given moment, the ovaries may respond to FSH, and this means that you may ovulate at random and unpredictable times. The estrogen, progesterone, FSH, and LH levels tend to be chaotic so that one day hormones are up, and the next they may be down. This chaos is the reason why symptoms can be so random and unpredictable. It is also important to remember that pregnancy can still occur during this time, so birth control is still recommended.

The follicles in the ovaries are key components to producing estrogen. As women get older, most follicles die off naturally, and some are used in menstruation or pregnancy. The remaining follicles (up to about 2,000) become less responsive. Menopause occurs when there are approximately 1,000 follicles remaining.

Although the current thinking is that women are born with a finite number of egg follicles (1 to 2 million), there is some new evidence that ovaries, at least in rats, have **stem cells** and may make new eggs up until menopause. More research is needed both to confirm these findings and to learn whether the process is similar in humans. But if this proves true in women, there are many implications for infertility treatment and for extending the reproductive period in women's lives.

8. How are the menstrual cycles of perimenopause similar to the menstrual cycles of puberty?

Perimenopause has been compared to puberty because the hormone levels and release of eggs can be

Luteinizing hormone

a hormone released from the pituitary gland that stimulates ovulation during the menstrual cycle. It also has a role in causing hot flashes.

Fallopian tubes

the slim straw-like tubes that lead from the ovaries to the top of either side of the uterus. The egg travels from the ovary through the fallopian tube to the uterus.

Corpus luteum

formed in the ovary as a result of the release of the mature egg.

Lutein

the yellowish pigment that gives the corpus luteum its yellowish color.

Stem cells

unspecialized cells that eventually develop into specialized cells, such as those found in the ovary.

equally chaotic in both of these normal life phases. The menstrual irregularities that occur during puberty—less frequent periods and cycles without ovulation—also occur during the menopause transition. The difference is that perimenopausal women tend to experience additional symptoms because their bodies have long been accustomed to the normal variations in hormones that occur with the menstrual cycle.

Once estrogen and progesterone decrease during perimenopause, symptoms occur because estrogen and progesterone receptor sites throughout the body respond to the erratic levels. Adolescent girls don't experience those symptoms because their bodies haven't become accustomed to the higher levels of hormones. Adolescent girls do experience some of the mood changes and sleep changes that are similar to the changes that women may experience during perimenopause.

Trina's comment:

Why do people want to treat menopause like it is a disease? We don't treat adolescents for hormone irregularities. Why should we treat older women for the same thing? Menopause is a natural part of life.

9. I thought that androgens were male hormones. Why do I need to know about them?

Adrenal glands

the two small endocrine glands located just above the kidneys. The adrenal glands secrete sex hormones, cortisol, and epinephrine.

Although men have more androgens than women, it is important to understand the role androgens play during menopause. Androgens are secreted by the ovaries and **adrenal glands**, and are converted throughout the body into estrogen. In women, androgens are important for reproductive function development, muscle development and strength, bone strength, and sexual function. They also play a role in determining the distribution of fat tissue throughout the body, and in providing energy and a sense of well-being. After menopause, androgens continue to be converted into estrogen by the adipose (fat) tissue. That's why women who are overweight and have more body fat (or **adipose tissue**) have higher levels of estrogen.

Androgens, especially **testosterone**, are believed to have an effect on sex drive, motivation for sex, and sensation. There are two types of testosterone, free and bound. Due to changes of aging, the amount of testosterone that is freely available (free testosterone) in a woman's body may decrease slightly. Only the free testosterone, comprising approximately 2% of the body's total testosterone, is available for use in the body tissues. In some cases the free testosterone will actually increase, occasionally leading to an increased interest in and enjoyment of sex during the perimenopausal years (see Question 24 regarding changes in sex drive with menopause). The ovary continues to produce androgens and testosterone even after menopause. Testosterone levels are lower in women who have had both of their ovaries removed.

Although estrogen also plays a role, testosterone is thought to play a greater role in maintaining sexual desire. Since estrogen levels decrease more rapidly than androgen levels, it means that there is a change in the ratio of estrogen to androgen. The change in this ratio helps explain some of the sexual problems women experience in postmenopause. (See Questions 67 and 89 about ways to help your sex drive.)

An Overview of Menopause

Adipose tissue

fat tissue. Androgens are changed to estrogen (estrone) in the adipose tissue.

Androgens

hormones secreted by the ovary and the adrenal gland that are important for libido, and balance with estrogen for sexual development.

Testosterone

a steroid hormone formed by the testes in males, and to a far lesser degree, by the ovary and adrenal glands in women. It is responsible for male characteristics such as a deep voice and facial hair, and is important for normal sexual development and function in women.

10. What is the average age of menopause?

The average age is 51. The range is generally from 48 to 55, but many normal women reach menopause at an age that falls out of this average range. Smokers tend to go through it about a year and a half earlier than the average non-smoking woman. And women who have had their uterus surgically removed also frequently experience menopause symptoms at an earlier age (see Question 14 about **hysterectomy**). There is some evidence that suggests that the age of a daughter's menopause will be about the same as her mother's. So, if your mother's menopause occurred at age 50, it is likely that your menopause will occur around age 50 as well. But of course, there are always exceptions!

The average age of 51 is computed based on all women, not just one racial or ethnic group, even though most of the data on menopause is based on the experiences of white women. African-American women tend to experience menopause slightly earlier than 51. Little data is currently available on the age of menopause for Asian or Latina women. But one study has shown that Latina or Hispanic women may experience menopause slightly earlier (0.4 years earlier), and Japanese-American women a little later (0.4 years later) than their Caucasian counterparts.

Having an early or late menopause could be associated with some different risks and benefits. Earlier menopause means you have fewer hassles with menstruation and freedom from the worry about pregnancy, but it is also associated with an increased risk for heart disease and **osteoporosis** due to the early loss of natural estrogen. Having a later menopause has some benefits and pitfalls, too. Later menopause means that you have

Hysterectomy

removal of the uterus.

Osteoporosis

a reduction in bone density that makes bone more fragile and susceptible to fractures.

been exposed to hormones for a longer period of time, which can possibly increase risks for hormone-linked cancers, but it also means that your increased risk for heart disease and osteoporosis is postponed.

11. How long can I expect to menstruate? Can I predict when I'll have my final menstrual period?

Menarche is the age at which you get your first menstrual period. Until about 200 years ago, menarche averaged around the age of 17. Now, the average age of menarche is about 13 years, but may be earlier among African-American teenagers, which means that women menstruate longer than they used to. This also means that the length of our **menstrual life** has increased.

Menarche
the first menstrual period.

Menstrual life is determined by subtracting the age of menarche (first menses) from the age at menopause, multiplying by 13 (the number of cycles per year), and then subtracting the months of pregnancies and months of breastfeeding. See Figure 7 for the formula.

Menstrual life
the number of menstrual periods in your lifetime.

Women from ancient societies had shorter menstrual lives. Women in ancient societies probably had about 100 menstrual cycles, whereas women today average about 450. Our ancestors had a later menarche, many more pregnancies, they breast fed their babies for longer periods, and died at a younger age than we currently do. Some have speculated that the food we eat today, such as meat from animals fed by food containing antibiotics and hormones, contributes to a younger menarche. But we really don't know for sure why girls get their first periods at a younger age.

Your menstrual life is calculated by multiplying the total number of years in which you menstruate by 13 (which is the number of cycles most women have in a year) and subtracting the total amount of time during your life in which your menstrual cycle was interrupted by pregnancy and breastfeeding.

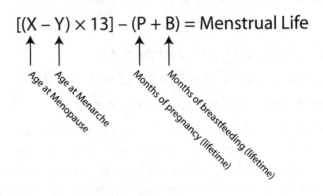

$$[(X - Y) \times 13] - (P + B) = \text{Menstrual Life}$$

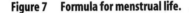

Figure 7   Formula for menstrual life.

The year of your menopause is *not* linked to your age at menarche. Common folklore and misperceptions say that if you menstruate early, you'll be done with menstruation early, but it doesn't work that way. However, if you are over 44 and have no periods for more than 60 days, or are having very irregular cycles, you are more likely to reach menopause in the next 4 years.

If you have reached the age of 51 without any symptoms of perimenopause, you are far more likely to have a shorter time leading up to your final menstrual period. Even though we know that most women experience menopause between the ages of 48 and 55, and that your mother's age at menopause may offer a clue, predicting when you will go through menopause is still tricky.

Madeline's comment:

I'm 54. I started menstruating when I was 10½. I was about 41 when I totally stopped my periods. One sister had a hysterectomy in her 30s so we don't know exactly when she would have hit menopause naturally. My younger sister stopped at age 38 and my mother was 45—she remembers because she was totally done just before my wedding day, and she always said that was a good date to remember!

12. What other circumstances can cause menopause?

Premature or early menopause is natural menopause but occurs in a woman who is less than 40 years old. Premature menopause is quite rare; only about 1% of the female population experiences this type of menopause. The reason for premature menopause is unknown.

Idiopathic ovarian insufficiency or **premature ovarian failure** is the loss of ovarian function (and therefore fertility) in a woman under the age of 40, resulting in menopause. It is usually associated with other health conditions such as autoimmune or genetic disorders, Addison's disease (a disorder of steroid hormone production), or hypothyroidism (low thyroid hormone production; see Question 47), and causes increased rates of osteoporosis (thinning of bone). See Questions 37–40. Premature ovarian failure can sometimes be temporary and is not exactly the same as premature menopause, which is permanent.

Amenorrhea (having no period for 3 months or more) that lasts for over one year is sometimes called **tempo-**

Premature or early menopause
permanent natural menopause occurring in a woman who is younger than 40 years of age.

Premature menopause is quite rare.

Idiopathic ovarian insufficiency or premature ovarian failure
the loss of ovarian function (and therefore fertility) in a woman under the age of 40, resulting in menopause. It is usually associated with other health conditions and can sometimes be temporary.

Amenorrhea
absence of menstruation for 3 months or more.

Temporary menopause

temporary loss of periods for over 1 year. Occurs when normal function of the ovary is interrupted either by medications, cancer treatments, stress, over-exercising, severe weight loss, or for unknown reasons.

Idiopathic

having no known cause.

Endometriosis

a painful condition characterized by the abnormal presence of endometrial tissue outside the uterus, such as on an ovary, the colon, or bladder.

Fibroid

a type of noncancerous tumor, also called leiomyomas, found in the uterus.

Induced menopause

permanent menopause that is not natural; can happen as a result of removal of the ovaries, chemotherapy, or radiation to the pelvis.

rary menopause, and happens when normal function of the ovary is interrupted. While this is referred to as temporary menopause, it is very different from true menopause because ovarian function and menstruation do return. We don't always know why it happens. It is often **idiopathic**, meaning without explanation. Temporary menopause can occur due to ovarian function suppression in athletes who exercise excessively, or with severe diet restriction as in persons with eating disorders. Once exercise is stopped or reduced, or a normal nutritional status is restored, ovarian function resumes, and menstrual periods return. Similarly, menses can be interrupted temporarily following some types of chemotherapy or pelvic radiation treatments, and in response to certain medications, such as GnRH analogues (usually used for severe **endometriosis** or **fibroids**), or unusually high doses of steroids. Temporary menopause is usually accompanied by menopausal symptoms, and is difficult to identify because it isn't certain if it is temporary until ovarian function and menstruation resume.

Induced menopause is permanent menopause that is not natural. It can be caused by removal of both ovaries (bilateral **oophorectomy**), disruption in normal ovarian function due to chemotherapy, or radiation to the pelvic region causing permanent disruption of ovarian function.

Surgical removal of the ovaries puts a woman into an abrupt, irreversible menopause, sometimes with very severe symptoms. Menopause caused by chemotherapy or radiation may happen after several months of treatment. Women may experience symptoms more gradually with chemotherapy- or radiation-induced menopause because the ovaries may not stop functioning as abruptly.

Jackie's comment:

I was about 38 when I was totally finished with periods. My sister was 41. Another sister had a hysterectomy in her 30s. My mother had her last period when she was 45, but her twin didn't hit menopause until she was 10 years older—boy was she jealous! I started having problems when I was about 37. I either had a heavy period or I'd go for a couple of months without having one. I started having hot flashes and mood swings. I told my husband that I thought I was going through menopause. I did some reading and really began to think it was possible that this was menopause. I made an appointment with my doctor, told her what was going on, and she said I was way too young but she would so some tests. Although we didn't think I was pregnant because I had my tubes tied when I was 28, we did a pregnancy test anyway. You just have to cover all the bases! My doctor called me back and said I was right—it was menopause. I was never given an explanation for the early menopause. But my feeling was, "Whew, I don't have to deal with my period ever again." I never saw it as losing my womanhood or anything like that. I said, "Yeah!" I actually saw it as a blessing.

13. What can I expect to experience if my menopause is induced?

Losing your fertility earlier than expected can be devastating. If you have been putting off pregnancy until you're older, losing your fertility can have a profound emotional effect. Some women choose to pursue

> **Oophorectomy**
> removal of one ovary. Bilateral oophorectomy is removal of both ovaries.

Losing your fertility can have a profound emotional effect.

An Overview of Menopause

options for preserving fertility, such as freezing some of their eggs prior to chemotherapy, or using donor eggs after their ovaries cease to produce eggs. However, not all women will have these options available to them—due to other health problems, cost, or lack of access to such services.

Those who experience induced menopause experience the same symptoms of natural menopause, but these symptoms can be very severe and may include more frequent hot flashes, increased sleeplessness, and more mood changes. The symptoms may be more severe because there's an early and sudden drop in hormone levels. Hormone production simply stops. Hormones do not fluctuate over time, and the body has no opportunity to grow accustomed to any of the changes in hormone levels.

Because estrogen has protective qualities for bone, there is a higher risk for osteoporosis in women with induced or early menopause. See Question 37 for a full discussion of the effect of menopause on bones. Likewise, because estrogen also has some protective effects on the heart and blood vessels, the risk for early **cardiovascular** disease increases. See Questions 44–46 for more information about heart disease and menopause.

Cardiovascular

relating to the heart or blood vessels.

14. What is a hysterectomy, and how does it affect menopause?

A hysterectomy is surgical removal of the uterus. Women may have a hysterectomy for the treatment of endometrial cancer and other conditions such as fibroids, excessive uterine bleeding, or **uterine prolapse**.

Uterine prolapse

when the uterus sits at a lower place in the abdominal cavity or slips into the vagina.

Many women mistakenly believe that the removal of their uterus puts them into instant menopause. This is incorrect. They will no longer menstruate and cannot support a pregnancy, but their ovaries are still producing all of the cyclic hormones. Since the uterus is not really part of the hormone cycle, its removal does not affect levels of estrogen, progesterone, FSH, LH, and GnRH. This leaves the HPO axis the way it was before the surgery.

So, if you have your uterus removed before you reach menopause, you will experience all of the same symptoms of perimenopause as you would if you still had your uterus. You will not, however, have irregular periods because you can no longer menstruate. Many women who have had their uterus removed do experience menopause at an earlier age, most likely due to a reduction in blood flow to the ovaries that often occurs following hysterectomy.

Removing the uterus and ovaries is called a **total hysterectomy** with a bilateral oophorectomy. If a woman is having a hysterectomy and oophorectomy, the fallopian tubes are removed as well (total hysterectomy with bilateral **salpingo-oophorectomy**). Following the surgical removal of the ovaries, unlike removal of the uterus alone, there is an immediate and sudden drop in hormone production. A woman whose ovaries have been removed may experience the abrupt onset of symptoms of menopause, and in some cases, the symptoms can be quite severe.

Total hysterectomy
although technically only refers to removal of the uterus, "total" is sometimes used to refer to removal of the uterus, ovaries, and fallopian tubes.

Salpingo-oophorectomy
removal of fallopian tubes and ovaries.

An Overview of Menopause

Emma's comment:

After the birth of my last child at age 39, my husband and I thought we better think of better ways to prevent pregnancy than counting days after a period and before the onset of another as to when I would be egg-free. I started taking birth control pills. When I was nearing 50, my husband needed hernia surgery, and his surgeon suggested that he have a vasectomy at the same time. He also suggested that this would allow me to go off the pill, because, I was told, I was too old to stay on the pill.

As soon as I stopped taking the pill, my periods became extremely heavy, most of the time lasting 10 days. I also started bleeding after intercourse. As if this was not enough, my emotions flared easily, yelling at the children, my husband, and the world in general, with copious tears mopped up with tissues and, some days, big paper towels.

My family doctor recommended a visit to my gynecologist, who in turn recommended a D & C. At this time I had missed no periods, and I had no hot flashes or headaches, which seemed to be the case with many of my friends. But maybe they didn't cry or shout as often as I did! What I lacked in hot flashes I probably got rid of in excess fluid by having crying fits.

After the D & C, the word was that there seemed to be some "precancerous cells" and we should keep an eye on it. A funny way of putting it really. Was I going to sit in a chair or on the sofa, or sit cross-legged in bed and watch for cancer? So rather than wait indefinitely, the surgery was scheduled for the summer when I wouldn't be teaching.

To my husband, I was very upbeat and went on about the wonders of no more worrying about having another child. We could chase each other all over our king-sized bed and not worry about a thing. Inside me was an entirely different scenario. I was convinced in my own mind that I would no longer be attractive physically, that I would be completely unable to have an orgasm, and I would have to learn how to fake an absolutely wonderful relationship with my husband. He, being a very quiet person, must have had his own doubts too, but never relayed them to me.

My surgeon took out the uterus but left my one ovary (I had the other removed when I was 20 because of a large ovarian cyst). He told me that menopause would come as less of a shock if I still had at least one ovary! After surgery I was overwhelmed again with the same pattern of up-and-down behavior, although it was mostly crying. Even seeing a sad news story on TV resulted in tears and tissue. The word "hysterical" has always seemed to me to go hand in hand with hysterectomy!

My doctor gave me some estrogen, and from then on I started to slowly come down this strange mountain I had been on for such a long time. The estrogen helped, but I did not like the soreness of my breasts and I felt I was getting more rotund than I wanted to be. So I weaned myself off the tablets, and started to lead a more normal life again. I was physically fit by the time school started in September. I became my old whirlwind self. Quite frankly, I was so busy getting my groove back, I didn't take the time to wonder if I was still attractive, or could enjoy the closeness of being a wife again. Somehow, it all evolved slowly. We became a couple again. I yelled a lot less and the tears seemed to dry up all on their own. And my concern about the hysterectomy was unfounded: Sex was wonderful and orgasms abounded.

Louanne's comment:

I had a hysterectomy when I was only 29. But the only time I actually miss my uterus is anytime I try to access the health care system for anything. The question, "date of your last menstrual period," clearly does not have a check mark for loss of uterus. Before menopause, it has to be a line for a date or a checkmark. But with no uterus, there's nothing to check. Since I was so young when I had my hysterectomy, people even ask me if I'm sure that I don't have a uterus— like the time I had such a bad urinary tract infection that I had clots in my urine, I was told that if I had clots, I must have my period. I miss my uterus more now at 46 then ever before mostly because I have no idea if or where I am in the menopause calendar... and no one seems to know definitively how to decide... I was never given any information when I had my uterus removed. I still have my ovaries but no one ever told me what to expect.

PART TWO

Experiencing the Symptoms of Menopause

What kind of symptoms can I expect to experience as I transition into menopause?

What is a hot flash?

What causes me to be so irritable and cry so easily?

Why do I seem to forget things more easily?

Why can't I get a good night's sleep?

More...

15. What types of symptoms can I expect to experience during perimenopause and postmenopause?

Every woman experiences menopause differently.

Every woman experiences menopause differently. You may experience a whole range of symptoms, or you may experience very few. Some symptoms will be very bothersome, and others quite manageable. The most common symptoms of menopause include hot flashes, sleep disturbances (often related to nighttime hot flashes and sweats), mood changes, and vaginal dryness.

Symptoms can range from mild to severe. There isn't an exact definition for severity of symptoms. Instead, it is based on how frequent and bothersome symptoms are for you. For example, having a few mild hot flashes in a day may not bother you, so your symptoms would be mild. If your hot flashes are mild and more frequent but you're bothered by sweating, your symptoms might be considered moderate. If you have profuse sweating with frequent hot flashes day and night, then your symptoms would generally be considered severe.

Prescription

an instruction from a licensed clinician, such as a physician, an advanced practice nurse, a midwife, or a physician's assistant, that provides for a medication or device to be issued by a pharmacy.

The usual approach for managing menopausal symptoms is to begin with lifestyle changes like diet and exercise, then add vitamins or minerals, and finally consider **prescription** or herbal therapies if symptoms cannot be managed effectively without them. See Parts 4 and 5 for information about managing menopausal symptoms.

See Table 1 (page 4) for a list of symptoms commonly experienced during perimenopause, the menopausal transition, and postmenopause.

Bridget's comment:

Why didn't someone tell me hot flashes were like this? I might have saved my money and moved to Antarctica or installed a walk-in freezer in my home and office. I never experienced childbirth firsthand, but puberty was a breeze compared with this maturational upheaval. I may be learning something, but so far I've no great insights to share, just a litany of premenopausal complaints. Menopause. They've got to be kidding. This ain't no pause. It's some sort of cataclysmic ending. I wonder how many women have endured all this sweat and steam and kept their mouths politely shut. Not me. I need to rant and rave.

16. What are hot flashes, and when do they happen?

Hot flashes, also called hot flushes, are generally described as a feeling of heat that starts at the top of the head and spreads throughout the body. Some women say that the feeling of heat starts at their center and moves outward, and some women report having the sense that they are about to have a hot flash.

Hot flashes that are accompanied by reddening of the skin, especially around the chest, head, and neck, are sometimes called hot flushes. You may also experience sweating, and in some cases, the sweating may be profuse. Women usually report that hot flashes are more bothersome at night, probably because their sleep is interrupted and not necessarily because they are worse than daytime flashes. Hot flashes that happen at night accompanied by profuse sweating are called "night sweats."

Women often report that hot flashes are their most bothersome symptom of menopause.

While most postmenopausal women report having hot flashes, they are most common in women who smoke or whose mothers had hot flashes. Women often report that hot flashes are their most bothersome symptom of menopause because they interfere not only with sleep, but activities of daily living and working. Whether you have had hot flashes while teaching your high school physics class or while sitting quietly at home, you may find them very distressing. Or, you may find that you're able to cope with the inconvenience and discomfort of hot flashes without seeking any specific treatment.

About one third of women won't have any hot flashes, another third will have mild to moderate hot flashes, and the remaining third will experience severe and frequent hot flashes. Mild hot flashes can just cause a feeling of warmth while very severe hot flashes can make you feel like you are really burning up one minute and then cold the next due to sweating and the rapid changes in core body temperature.

Hot flashes may occur only once or twice a day, or as often as every few minutes. They may last for a few seconds or for several minutes or more. Women are more likely to experience hot flashes during postmenopause than they are during perimenopause.

Once they reach menopause, most women will have hot flashes for an average of 7 years. A smaller group of women will experience hot flashes for up to 20 years, and in some cases even longer. For information on managing your hot flashes, see Parts 4 and 5.

Bridget's comment:

Vague apprehension gives way to full-blown queasiness then escalates to breathlessness. The word "suffocating" crosses my mind. Waves of prickling warmth creep across my scalp and down my forehead, neck, and chest. My heart starts to pound. I actually feel steam rising through my clothes. Suddenly, my pores sprout rivers of sweat, which drip down the sides of my face, my chest, and even down my arms and legs. Water droplets collect on the inside of my glasses. If I'm alone, I swear, fan myself like mad, and strip away layers of clothing. When the sensation passes, I'm cold, clammy, and cranky, and after two or three of these an hour, I'm ready for the wringer.

17. Why do hot flashes occur?

Although hot flashes are not physically harmful to you and do not pose a health hazard, there may be physiologic reasons why they occur. For one thing, there is a measurable change in the skin surface temperature that accompanies a hot flash, and the core body temperature is lower after the hot flash. Some women feel cold after the hot flash subsides, especially if it is accompanied by sweating. During a normal menstrual cycle, as FSH and LH levels increase, estrogen levels also increase. But that doesn't always happen in perimenopause. Sometimes there is a sudden rise in luteinizing hormone (LH) without a corresponding increase in estrogen. This coincides with the stimulation of the **vasomotor** cells in the brain and the release of substances that make the peripheral blood vessels dilate, causing a hot flash.

The consistently lower levels of estrogen found during postmenopause are partly responsible for causing hot

Vasomotor

the part of the brain that regulates dilation and constriction of blood vessels. Vasomotor symptoms usually include hot flashes and night sweats.

flashes to occur as well. Taking estrogen does reduce the frequency and severity of hot flashes in many women. In fact, estrogen is the single most effective treatment for hot flashes (see Part 5, Hormone therapy and Other Options).

Alcohol, caffeine, and spicy foods can precipitate hot flashes, as can walking from a cold room to a hot one. Stress can also be a trigger for hot flashes.

Hot flashes are known to be more severe and last longer in women who have had their ovaries removed. Whether or not you still have your ovaries, there is no way to predict how many months or years you will experience hot flashes. Smokers and obese women (those with a body mass index or BMI of >30; see Question 36) also have more severe hot flashes and may have more frequent flashes as well.

You may experience **palpitations** (rapid, sometimes irregular heartbeat) or a **panic attack** during a hot flash. Sometimes the feeling that you are going to have a hot flash can actually bring on a panic attack in those who have had them before.

There are some ethnic differences in the way women report hot flashes and night sweats. In the SWAN (Study of Women's Health Across the Nation) Study, African-American women were most likely to report having hot flashes and/or night sweats, followed by Hispanic women, Caucasian women, and Asian women.

Hot flashes can also occur due to other health problems such as diabetes, high blood pressure, and **hyperthyroidism** (overproduction of thyroid hormone). People who take niacin for management of high cho-

Hormone therapy

an umbrella term that describes the use of estrogen, progesterone, or some combination of the two, and sometimes testosterone, to treat the symptoms of menopause.

Palpitations

abnormally fast or irregular heartbeats.

Panic attack

sudden onset of intense apprehension, fear, or impending doom accompanied by physical symptoms such as nausea, sweating, and heart palpitations.

Hyperthyroidism

overproduction of thyroid hormone.

lesterol, and men who are taking hormones for the treatment of prostate cancer may also have hot flashes. See Question 53 about other medical conditions that can cause symptoms like those of menopause.

Bridget's comment:

When the night sweats started one August four years ago, I thought I had AIDS or TB. It took me a while to figure out what was really happening. I was too young for menopause. Back then, my thermostat went out of whack for only three or four weeks at a time. I felt like a furnace in overdrive until my cycle kicked back in again. Maybe the goddess of fertility is loathe to give up on us childless women. Hot flashes might be her signaling system as she tries to maneuver those last few aging eggs into a receiving position.

18. My periods are so irregular. Sometimes they are 3 weeks apart and sometimes 6 weeks apart. I've recently been bleeding for several weeks. Is that normal?

Almost every woman who has not had her uterus removed will experience irregular menstrual periods. You can definitely expect changes in your menstrual pattern during perimenopause. The irregularity of your periods results from fewer cycles with ovulation, and irregular estrogen and progesterone levels. Heavier women and older women are most likely to experience menstrual irregularities. Women of Chinese or Japanese descent may also experience irregularities more often than other women.

Since irregular periods are the most common sign of perimenopause, you can expect to experience changes in one or all of the following: quantity of menstrual bleeding, duration of your period, and time between periods. This means that your periods could become heavier, lighter, shorter, longer, and may change from month to month. They could also become less frequent, more frequent, or you may stop menstruating for several months at a time. Sometimes, after several weeks or months without a period, the menstrual flow can be brown.

This is not to say that all menstrual irregularity is normal, or that you can always attribute it to perimenopause. Once you begin to notice irregularity, it's a good idea to keep a diary of your periods. This will help your clinician determine the cause of the irregularity. If you miss a period, develop heavier bleeding, bleed 2 days longer than usual, spot between periods, or bleed after intercourse, it is important to contact your clinician because abnormal bleeding can also be caused by fibroids, endometriosis, certain cancers, blood disorders, thyroid problems, birth control pills, pregnancy, and hormone imbalances not related to perimenopause. See Table 2 for an overview of different menstrual bleeding irregularities.

Heavy bleeding is defined as passing more than about 2½ ounces of menstrual blood (average blood loss is about 1 ounce). But it's very difficult to measure. So, if you are using many extra pads or tampons in a day, or passing frequent and/or large clots, you have heavy bleeding and should contact your clinician. Sometimes very heavy bleeding is severe enough to cause **iron deficiency anemia**. Your clinician may want to evaluate the bleeding by doing an **ultrasound** or **biopsy** of

Iron deficiency anemia

blood disorder characterized by loss of oxygen-carrying blood cells either by inadequate iron intake or by loss of blood.

Ultrasound

use of high-frequency sound waves to visualize organs of the body.

Biopsy

a piece of tissue removed from the body and examined for abnormalities.

Table 2   Menstrual Bleeding Irregularities

Medical Term	Definition
Amenorrhea	Absence of or missed period (usually at least 3 cycles)
Dysmenorrhea	Painful menstruation
Intermenstrual bleeding	Bleeding between periods
Menorrhagia	Abnormally heavy or long periods
Metrorrhagia	Irregular bleeding between periods
Oligomenorrhea	Light bleeding or infrequent periods (>35 days apart)
Premenstrual bleeding	Spotting or light bleeding before regular period

the uterine lining, and may prescribe progestin or estrogen depending on how long you have been bleeding and how heavy the bleeding is.

Persistent bleeding is usually related to an overgrowth of the uterine lining that happens when the ratio of estrogen to progesterone produced by the body is out of balance. When the ratio is out of balance the uterine lining continues to build up, but doesn't shed properly in the normal monthly period. When this happens, bleeding can sometimes persist for 2 to 3 weeks. If this occurs, your clinician will examine you and may order an ultrasound or biopsy. Usually you would be prescribed progestin pills. Progestin pills will stabilize the uterine lining so the bleeding stops, usually within a few days. After you stop taking the progestin pills, you will likely get a heavy "withdrawal" bleed or period, which usually lasts 5 to 7 days, but is much heavier than a normal period.

Experiencing the Symptoms of Menopause

Madeline's comment:

For about four years, my periods were on and off. I'd go for a couple of months without one and then they'd start right up again. One of the last periods I had was so painful that I told myself that if I had another period like that one, I would go to the emergency room. I had one last period that was just spotting and then I was really done!

19. What causes me to feel irritable and cry more easily?

The bad news is that irritability and crying for no apparent reason happen more frequently during perimenopause. The good news is that mood swings are less common once you reach menopause and after.

It's difficult to pinpoint the exact reason for moodiness during perimenopause, but it's probably related to unexpected and unpredictable shifts in hormone levels, which are often dramatically different than the monthly fluctuations a woman becomes used to during a normal menstrual cycle. Some mood changes, especially irritability, difficulty concentrating, and fatigue, may be more strongly linked to sleep disturbances. Stress can also add to irritability (see Question 42).

Some women can't sleep because of their hot flashes, which brings on fatigue, mood swings, irritability, and less ability to cope during waking hours. The lack of sleep can also interfere with memory and **cognitive** abilities (see Question 31). The stress that many women feel due to moodiness and memory changes can itself increase the frequency and severity of hot flashes, creating a circular pattern of hot flashes caus-

Cognitive

pertaining to the areas of the brain that control reasoning, judgment, knowing, imagining, and memory.

ing sleep disturbances, and the stress related to lack of sleep resulting in increased hot flashes, and again, more fatigue.

Women who have already experienced depression are more likely to become depressed once they start perimenopause. Women who also have had severe mood changes associated with their menstrual periods may experience more mood swings during perimenopause. Many women report a worsening of their PMS symptoms during perimenopause. But if you've never been depressed and you haven't had big mood changes around your periods, that doesn't mean that you won't have mood changes during perimenopause. Depression affects about three times as many women in perimenopause as it does prior to that time.

You may be having mood changes that are totally unrelated to perimenopause. Untreated depression, medications, medical conditions such as thyroid disorders, nutritional deficiencies, or stressful life events may also cause mood changes. See Question 41, which addresses depression and the need for getting help from a mental health professional.

Bridget's comment:

Strangely enough, not only does the sweat drip, the tears flow as well. The radio does it for me these days—a song, a commercial, the slightest hint of emotion in a news story and I'm all choked up. I read a letter, a poem, a sad or happy novel, the greeting on a card and I swoon. I'm careful to keep this to myself, though. No one would believe I struggle to suppress sobs through AT&T commercials.

Madeline's comment:

Weepy? I felt just like a pre-teen when you're so emotional. I remember crying over commercials on TV. I also remember my youngest daughter was around 12 or 13 at the time. She was angry at me and I was angry at her. She started crying and I started crying. She sobbed, "I don't know why I'm crying!" And I sobbed right back, "I don't know why either!" I remember that old teenage feeling—nobody understands me! I felt like I was 13 and my mother was being mean. It was just awful and I couldn't help myself— the emotions are just that close to the edge. Then one day, it just dawned on me, "Oh, this is menopause!" Once I finally knew what I was feeling, it did help me understand—it didn't always make it better but it did help to know what it was!

20. Why do I forget things more easily?

You probably feel like you're the only one who can't remember where the car keys are or the five things you had to buy at the grocery store. But forgetfulness and lack of concentration are common occurrences during midlife and as you approach menopause.

Progesterone, androgens, and especially estrogen have receptors in the brain, and are believed to affect learning and memory. When you are going through perimenopause and postmenopause, these brain receptors are likely to respond in a negative way to rapidly changing and lower levels of hormones.

Stressor

anything that causes stress.

Fatigue, moodiness, poor sleep, midlife **stressors**, and even physical symptoms from illness can affect your ability to concentrate, focus, and therefore, to remember. If you are having difficulty concentrating, you will have a hard time learning new things and remembering things.

All aspects of **cognition** (reasoning, concentration, memory, spatial relationships) decrease with age in men and women. Because estrogen has been linked to brain function, it was believed that estrogen therapy would decrease the risk of getting **Alzheimer's**. But research results testing this theory have been controversial (see Questions 75 and 78 about hormone therapy). It is not known whether the estrogen changes that accompany perimenopause and menopause cause the cognitive changes that so many women experience. Sleep loss that frequently results from nighttime hot flashes definitely does interfere with memory and concentration, but may not fully explain cognitive changes in all women.

So, if you're having difficulty remembering things, it's partly because of age, partly because of hormones, and partly because of poor sleep and midlife events.

Trina's comment:

You get up to do something and you don't remember what you got up to do. And then you put something down and you don't remember where, and you can't even blame anybody. It's so embarrassing. And it's so funny too, because you're talking and all of a sudden, you lose it and can't remember what you were going to say. Then you're like... wait a minute, I know I'm not crazy!

21. My breasts are quite tender, even between my periods. Is that normal?

Breast tenderness is a common symptom during perimenopause and is usually associated with the rise in hormones just before you get your period. Breast tenderness occurs at other times than just before your periods because of the hormonal chaos that is associated

Cognition

mental processes that are related to knowledge gathering, judgment, reasoning, imagining, and memory.

Alzheimer's

degenerative brain disorder that gradually causes disorientation, confusion, and memory loss.

with perimenopause. Estrogen and progesterone levels can be high both before periods and at other times, causing you to have tender breasts more frequently.

Breast tenderness during postmenopause is uncommon except when a woman takes hormone therapy (see Questions 78 and 83 about the side effects of hormone therapy, and how to manage those side effects).

Women who have breast lumps, nipple discharge, or irregularities or thickening of the breast tissue should seek help from their clinician as soon as possible.

Although some women may immediately leap to the conclusion that breast tenderness means a diagnosis of cancer, breast cancer rarely presents with tenderness or soreness. But it can happen, so if your breast tenderness is persistent or concerns you, you should see your clinician. Women who have breast lumps, nipple discharge, or irregularities or thickening of the breast tissue should seek help from their clinician as soon as possible. See Question 43 about breast cancer.

22. Why do I gain weight more easily during menopause?

Your weight gain is more likely related to normal aging changes and your lifestyle rather than menopause itself.

Studies have shown that women in the menopausal transition gain an average of 5 pounds. This weight gain was often attributed to the hormone therapy used to treat menopausal symptoms. There is no scientific evidence, however, that weight gain during menopause has anything to do with a decrease in your estrogen levels or the use of hormone therapy.

Despite the fact that you have gained weight around the time of menopause, your weight gain is more likely related to normal aging changes and your lifestyle rather than menopause itself.

It's normal to lose some lean body mass (muscle) as we age. It is also normal for body fat to accumulate as we age. The distribution of fat also changes during menopause. When you were premenopausal, you had a tendency to put on fat around your buttocks and your thighs. If you're postmenopausal, you're more likely to see fat accumulate around your middle.

In order to maintain your premenopausal weight, you must eat fewer calories and burn more calories. It's as simple as that. Eat less and exercise more. Because we are naturally more sedentary as we age, have a slower metabolism, and have greater fat stores, we must decrease our food intake and increase our activity to avoid gaining weight. But it isn't easy! One pound equals 3,500 calories, and it isn't easy to trim that much out of your usual diet. That's why exercise is so important. The more you move, the more calories you use.

Eat less and exercise more.

Trina's comment:

For me it is the weight. That's my number one concern. I just keep gaining, and it's around my middle. Some days I think I look like I am pregnant again! Except that it is spread all around. I have been dieting and trying to exercise, but it doesn't seem to help. I feel so frustrated...

Clarissa's comment:

I was gaining weight. I couldn't seem to control it. So I went to see my nurse practitioner and she explained about the changes in metabolism, that my body uses food differently now, and that I need to make even bigger changes just to break even—that's not even talking about losing. So now I am exercising to boost my metabolism, and she said it is healthy for my heart and bones too. And I am watching what I eat, not just fewer calories, but healthier, more vegetables and less fat—it's working, but it is really slow.

23. I'm uncomfortable even when I sit. Sex is also very painful now that I've hit menopause. Is that normal?

Sometimes vaginal dryness in postmenopause can be so severe that women have trouble sitting comfortably. The friction between the dry walls of the vaginal can be quite painful, and can occur during normal activities or during complete inactivity. Since all women will experience changes in their urinary and vaginal tracts (**urogenital** changes) as a result of low estrogen levels in postmenopause, this is a very common problem. Some women do not find the changes bothersome; others require treatment (see Question 66 and 75 about treating vaginal dryness). The dryness can make sexual activity very painful (**dyspareunia**), and continued pain with intercourse can definitely reduce the desire to have sex.

Dryness is not the only vaginal problem related to menopause. Itching and irritation of the vaginal and urethral openings (see Figure 8 showing female anatomy) can also occur as a result of low levels of estrogen. You may be bothered by **vaginal discharge** accompanied by redness, itching, and irritation of the vagina (**vaginitis**). Discharge may or may not require treatment, but should be evaluated. It may be a normal response to decreased estrogen and friction. It may require treatment and can become recurrent. You should not assume that vaginitis or discharge is a nor-

Urogenital

relating to the urinary and the reproductive systems, especially the vagina in women (synonymous with genitourinary).

Dyspareunia

pain with sexual intercourse.

Vaginal discharge

substance that comes out of the vagina that results from normal mucous production, infection, hormones, overgrowth of normal vaginal bacteria, allergies, irritations, menstrual blood flow, or cancer.

Vaginitis

inflammation of the vagina.

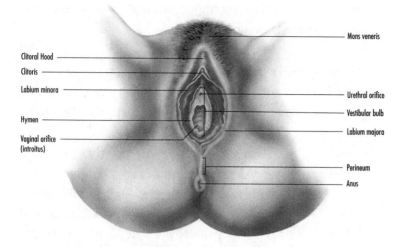

Clitoral Hood

Clitoris

Labium minora

Hymen

Vaginal orifice
(introitus)

Mons veneris

Urethral orifice

Vestibular bulb

Labium majora

Perineum

Anus

Figure 8   Female anatomy (external view of perineum).

mal result of low estrogen levels. Vaginitis with or
without discharge can be caused by vaginal infection
such as yeast, **trichomoniasis**, or overgrowth of normal bacteria; medications such as antibiotics; sexual
transmitted infections; allergic and chemical reactions
to soaps, bubble baths, spermicidal jellies, condoms,
feminine hygiene sprays, or deodorant tampons or
pads; **douching**; irritation from leaving tampons or
birth control devices such as diaphragms in too long;
skin conditions such as eczema; Crohn's disease; injury
to pelvic nerves leading to persistent pain; or even a
sensitivity to a male partner's semen.

During your postmenopause years, you can become
more sensitive to fragrances and chemicals that you've
always used or been around. As you get older, even toilet paper and familiar hygiene products can become
irritating to you. Douching is discouraged not only
because of this increased chemical sensitivity, but

Trichomoniasis

vaginal inflammation
caused by an organ-
ism called *Tri-
chomonas vaginalis*.
It is usually transmit-
ted during sex.

Douching

the act of using water
mixed with medica-
tion or cleansing
agent with the intent
of hygiene or
treatment of the
vagina.

*You can
become more
sensitive to
fragrances and
chemicals that
you've always
used or been
around.*

45

because it tends to remove normal vaginal bacteria which keeps the vagina healthy.

Some women can become very sensitive to semen as they age. There is an increasing difference between the acidity of the semen and the vagina, causing further irritation.

Low levels of estrogen contribute to the increased fragility of the vagina, meaning the vagina is easily injured, even with normal activities such as inserting a tampon or diaphragm. In postmenopause, it is not uncommon for women to bleed a little after penetration during sex. This may simply indicate that you need to use more **lubrication**. But you should never assume that bleeding after intercourse is normal until you have talked with your clinician.

Trina's comment:

So, you know, I used to really enjoy sex, but now it just plain hurts. I even hurt sometimes when I am just sitting here minding my own business. So how am I supposed to get in the mood when I know it's going to hurt? My man, he doesn't get it at all, sometimes he gets annoyed about it. I don't like using the jelly, but what can I do? Who knew that this menopause thing could mess up so many areas of my life?

24. How will menopause affect my sex drive?

It's not your imagination if you are having more difficulty becoming aroused and reaching orgasm, or if you are less interested in sex as you approach menopause and after. Changes around sexual health occur as a result of both the normal aging process and the variation in hormones.

Lubrication

using a water-soluble substance to make sexual intercourse more comfortable if normal vaginal lubrication isn't possible either because of lack of arousal or because of vaginal atrophy.

Women in perimenopause report concerns with decreased sexual satisfaction, desire, and arousal; inadequate lubrication; more difficulty reaching orgasm; and more discomfort during intercourse. All of these symptoms occur more frequently after menopause. Lower estrogen levels have definitely been associated with vaginal dryness, pain with intercourse, and pain with vaginal penetration.

Some sexual changes are related to the normal aging process. After menopause, it generally takes longer to become lubricated. There is also less lubrication fluid, a decrease in the elasticity of the vagina, and the tissue around the clitoris shrinks. The vaginal walls become thinner and paler, and are more easily injured with normal sexual activities. Vaginal changes also make you more susceptible to vaginal infections.

Some sexual changes are related to the normal aging process.

While you may experience some negative symptoms, the postmenopausal time can also alleviate some of the stresses associated with having sex. For example, menopause frees women from the fear of pregnancy. In addition, if your children are older, they are less likely to interrupt you, and you may have more time to spend pampering yourself and getting into the mood for intimacy with your partner.

Some medications may interfere with sex drive and achieving orgasm. For example, some antidepressants used for the treatment of hot flashes or depression may cause a decreased desire for sex, as well as difficulty having an orgasm. Medications for controlling blood pressure and cholesterol can also have adverse effects on your sex life. If you have recently started taking a new medication and you are experiencing new sexual problems, you should consult your clinician.

For women, sex is heavily affected by emotion. The task of getting the mind interested in sex, and the body physically aroused for sex, becomes more difficult with age. Don't be surprised if you need more romance and foreplay to enjoy sex with your partner, who is likely to be experiencing changes related to age as well.

Dissatisfaction with your sex life becomes its own negative feedback system: If sex is not satisfying or is uncomfortable, you can expect to become increasingly uninterested in it. But you don't have to tolerate a life without sex when you approach menopause. Management of sexual problems experienced during the menopausal transition and after is addressed in Questions 66, 67, and 89.

25. What kind of urinary changes can I expect during menopause?

The two major urinary changes you may experience during postmenopause are incontinence and infection, neither of which are normal aspects of aging or menopause. Both should be discussed with your clinician. Urinary incontinence (involuntary leakage or dribbling of urine) occurs in 10 to 30% of women aged 50 to 64, compared to only 1 to 5% of men the same age. There is a connection between the normal changes of aging and the hormonal changes of menopause that makes incontinence more likely for women.

Urinary infection, which can make incontinence worse, can be linked to the low estrogen levels of postmenopause. Typical symptoms of urinary infection include urgency to urinate, frequent urination, and burning with urination. Foul smelling or cloudy urine should be evaluated for possible infection as well, even if the other symptoms are not present. Some women experience recurrent urinary infections that require ongoing medical monitoring and treatment. If you suddenly develop incontinence and have bad smelling urine, it is possible that urgency from infection has caused your incontinence.

Normal urination requires coordination between your nervous system and bladder muscles. Your nervous system tells your bladder to "hold it" and to voluntarily release the urine when you're ready to do so. The nervous system assists with the function of the smooth muscle opening of the bladder (sphincter), allowing release of the urine into the urethra, and causes the bladder muscle to contract giving you the urge to urinate. There are estrogen receptors in both the urethra (the tube-like structure carrying urine from the bladder to the outside) and the bladder. As estrogen levels decline, muscle control and nerve function decline for both the bladder muscle and the bladder sphincter. These changes result in the need for more frequent urination, sudden urges to urinate, nighttime urination, and sometimes urine leakage with heavy lifting, or after coughing or sneezing.

26. What is incontinence, and how is it related to menopause?

There are three main kinds of urinary incontinence: urge, stress, and mixed. Urge incontinence increases with the number of years into postmenopause and happens when the main muscle of the bladder gets irritated and starts to contract, giving you the urge to urinate. The contraction can be strong enough to cause urine to leak out. Stress incontinence occurs more frequently during perimenopause, and happens when the bladder sphincter is unable to stay closed against abdominal pressure caused by coughing, lifting, sneezing, or exercising. The pressure pushes on the sphincter, which doesn't have the ability to stay closed, allowing urine to leak out. Mixed incontinence is the more common type and is a combination of both urge and stress.

Urinary incontinence is not an automatic byproduct of aging, but there are definite changes related to age that can affect normal urination:

- There's an increase in activity of the bladder muscle, meaning that it can get irritated and activated more easily and at inappropriate times, causing the urge to urinate or urine leakage.
- There's a decreased ability to "hold it" because of decreased muscle strength over time.
- There is an increase in urine flow because the muscles relax, opening up the bladder more quickly.
- There is an increase in residual urine (the amount of urine left in the bladder once you have finished urinating).
- The lower levels of estrogen during postmenopause cause shrinkage and decreased elasticity of the urethra.
- There is an increase in the amount of fluid sent to your kidneys when you are lying down, causing you to need to use the bathroom more frequently during the night.

There are many factors that increase the likelihood of developing incontinence:

- Low levels of estrogen
- Obesity

- Activities that increase abdominal pressure such as exercise or heavy lifting
- Certain medical conditions such as diabetes, congestive heart failure, **chronic obstructive pulmonary disease** (COPD), stroke, **Parkinson's** disease
- Depression
- Surgery or radiation of the genital or urinary system
- Pregnancy (vaginal delivery, especially of large babies with or without **episiotomy,** or the use of forceps during delivery that could have damaged muscles or nerves), surgery, or other trauma to the pelvic muscles or nerves
- Impaired mobility (difficulty getting to the bathroom fast enough)
- Certain medications such as tranquilizers or **diuretics**
- Constipation or fecal (stool) incontinence
- Urinary tract infections
- Irritated bladder from cigarette smoking or excessive alcohol or caffeine ingestion

Chronic obstructive pulmonary disease

a chronic lung disease that causes slowed or difficult breathing, wheezing, and increased mucous.

Parkinson's

a brain disorder characterized by abnormal movements, tremors, weakness, and sometimes paralysis. Usually affects people 50 years of age or older.

Episiotomy

incision made in the perineum to ease delivery of a baby.

Diuretic

substance or medication that causes an increase in urine excretion. Caffeine is an example of a naturally occurring mild diuretic.

Donna's comment:

Sometimes I barely make it to the bathroom, it's embarrassing. Sometimes the kids want to keep going, but I am the one who has to know where every bathroom is now. It just comes over me, it's like I have to go this second, and there really isn't any warning. I have a hard time holding it, so I avoid situations where I can't get to a bathroom—like I don't go to the kids' soccer games anymore, and I used to really enjoy them.

Sarah's comment:

The "water works" started—I couldn't sneeze without crossing my legs, couldn't exercise without leaking, couldn't take long walks without leaking, etc. Okay, you finally stop having your periods and think, WOW, no more tampons or pads—WRONG. Now it's even worse—you're wearing pads all the time—and big and bulkier ones—ugh. Try carrying these in a small purse!

27. I've always had migraines and was told they might disappear when I get to menopause. Is that true?

Women who have had headaches associated with their menstrual periods may have an increase in headaches during perimenopause caused by the erratically high levels of estrogen. But approximately two thirds of women who have experienced menstrual migraines will no longer have migraines once they are in postmenopause because of consistently lower levels of estrogen.

If you are using birth control pills, whether you're in perimenopause or not, headaches may occur during the **placebo** week (the week you are not taking estrogen or progesterone) and may be more severe if you are in perimenopause.

Tension headaches tend to affect women more often than men, and although not directly related to hormone changes, they are clearly associated with the stresses often experienced at midlife. The tension headache is often described as the feeling of a rubber band being tightened around the head, wearing a hat that is too tight, or a feeling of having the head squeezed on both sides. Tension headaches can last from 30 minutes to 7 days.

Cluster headaches affect men more than women, and can last up to 3 months. The severe pain of this type of

Placebo

an inactive substance that contains no medication or active ingredient to be given to participants in a clinical trial to determine the effectiveness of a particular medication or substance.

headache is usually behind one eye, often causing watering of the eye or severe facial pain.

Migraine headaches occur most frequently in women 25 to 55 years of age, and produce a moderate to severe throbbing, usually on one side of the head. Nausea, vomiting, and sensitivity to light, motion, and noise can persist for up to 72 hours. Sometimes an aura, which is often a visual change, precedes the migraine by about 1 hour.

Headaches must be evaluated by your clinician, particularly if they are new, if they increase from the usual severity, or if they are accompanied by stiff neck, numbness, tingling, weakness, dizziness, vision or hearing changes, or lack of coordination. Such headaches can be a symptom of infection, cardiovascular or neurological conditions, or cancer. Other causes for headaches can be sinusitis, allergies, colds, dental problems, and/or hangover from a night of partying.

Eliminating certain **triggers** can help you reduce the frequency of your headaches. Common headache triggers include alcohol; caffeine; foods that contain tyramine such as yogurt, sour cream, red wine, chocolate, and aged cheese; foods with nitrites such as bacon and hot dogs; and foods that contain MSG (**monosodium glutamate**), such as frozen foods or food from a Chinese restaurant. Other triggers include fasting or skipping meals; not drinking enough water; getting too much or too little sleep; stress or anxiety; environmental factors such as loud noises, changes in air pressure, breathing perfume, or bright lights; and hormone changes or therapy.

Triggers

foods, substances, or activities that prompt a certain response in the body.

Monosodium glutamate

a chemical substance used for seasoning food.

Zoe's comment:

I had terrible migraines starting in my 30s. I would get them right around ovulation and again right before my period would start. I wouldn't just get stabbing pain on one side of my head. The left side of my face would also droop. Sometimes I would see blurry and wavy lines and then my left eye pupil would dilate. I took many different medications, but the best cure seems to be menopause! I was told by my doctor almost 20 years ago that the migraines, although very difficult to treat then, would eventually get better when my hormones changed. He was right. I have not had a bad headache for months.

28. Sometimes I feel like my heart is going to jump out of my chest because it's beating so hard and fast. It's never done that before. Is that normal?

During a hot flash, you may feel like your heart is beating harder and out of control, or skipping beats (palpitations). The increased heart rate during a hot flash is actually a normal response by the heart to a change in body temperature.

There is some evidence that low levels of estrogen during postmenopause change the electrical activity of the heart, causing more palpitations. Stress, anxiety, and panic disorder can cause palpitations as well. Thyroid disease can cause palpitations and an overall increase or decrease in your resting heart rate. Cardiac arrhythmias, which are abnormal heart rhythms, do increase as women age, however, palpitations alone are not usually associated with heart disease. See Questions 44–46 concerning heart disease.

While palpitations associated with the menopausal transition are usually innocent and do not damage the heart, it is wise to discuss your palpitations with your clinician, especially if they are accompanied by shortness of breath, nausea, sweating without hot flashes, chest discomfort, or decreased tolerance for exertion or exercise.

Salt, medications such as pseudoephedrine (Sudafed) for colds, alcohol, smoking, fatigue, and caffeine can increase the occurrence of palpitations.

29. My joints ache. Am I just getting old, or is this part of menopause?

While many midlife women experience joint discomfort or pain during the menopause years, a definite link to menopause has not been made. Joint pain is an especially common symptom for midlife Asian women. The most common form of arthritis, **osteoarthritis**, affects more women after menopause because it's more common as we age, and is generally caused by normal "wear and tear" and inflammation. In general, joint pain will affect those who are less active because inactivity decreases strength and function of both muscles and joints. If muscles become weak, they cannot support joints, causing more wear and tear, and eventually more aches and pains. Obesity is a risk factor for developing osteoarthritis because of the stress put on the joints by excess weight.

Rheumatoid arthritis (RA), another cause of joint pain, is more common in women than men. Unlike osteoarthritis, RA is often accompanied by mild fever, joint pain, joint swelling, and fatigue. Rheumatoid arthritis is usually first diagnosed in women 35 to 50

Osteoarthritis
inflammation and stiffness of the joints that usually occurs in older persons as a result of deterioration of the cartilage around the joints.

Rheumatoid arthritis
a form of joint inflammation and stiffness that affects women more than men, and usually starts at an earlier age than osteoarthritis. The joints can later become deformed and cause considerable disability.

years of age. It's currently speculated that sex hormones, particularly estrogen, do have a role in immunity, which means that certain diseases like RA could be affected by changes in hormone levels.

30. My eyes tend to feel itchy and dry. Why is that?

It is common for your eyes to become itchy, dry, and even swollen beginning in perimenopause and continuing into postmenopause. Contact lenses can be bothersome, and some women will not be able to continue wearing contacts because of their dry eyes. If you have had refractive surgery to correct nearsightedness, you are more likely to develop dry eyes.

It is common for your eyes to become itchy, dry, and even swollen beginning in perimenopause and continuing into post–menopause.

Eye changes reported after menopause include dryness, pressure, blurred vision, intolerance to light and cold, increased or decreased tear and mucous production, tired eyes, burning, swollen or reddened eyelids, and scratchiness. Eye symptoms can also be caused by infection, blocked eye ducts, or connective tissue or immune diseases, so you should have symptoms evaluated before just chalking them up to menopause.

The need for reading glasses usually begins after age 40 in both men and women, and is unrelated to hormones. There is some evidence that estrogen taken during postmenopause may have a protective effect with regard to the development of **cataracts**.

Cataracts

a cloudy lens of the eye that leads to vision problems and if untreated can lead to blindness. Is usually surgically corrected.

Trina's comment:

It's so weird, everything is dry, even my eyes. Sometimes they feel like they have sandpaper in them. I can't close them without it hurting. It's like the tears just dried up, they don't come anymore—even if I cry they are dry. I have to use moisture drops but they only help for a little while. The moisture ointment is better, but sometimes it makes my vision blurry.

31. Why can't I get a good night's sleep?

It's not entirely accurate to blame lack of sleep on peri-menopause. Many components are important for a good night's sleep. Normal aging, illnesses and stress, lifestyle issues, and menopausal symptoms can all contribute to a bad night's sleep.

Before blaming sleeplessness on your hormones, you will want to have a look at your lifestyle, such as lack of exercise or exercising right before bedtime, eating before bedtime, drinking alcohol or caffeine, and taking drugs that have a stimulant effect.

Other reasons for sleep disturbances besides decreasing estrogen levels can include stress, depression, excessive napping, having a restless sleep partner, illness such as anemia and thyroid disease, uncomfortable sleep accommodations, and too much activity close to bedtime. Still other factors might include noise, a partner who snores, a room that is too hot, or worries about health, work, children, or parents. There are many factors that can interfere with a good night's sleep.

Sleep can clearly be disturbed by hot flashes or night sweats. Some women awaken because they're just hot, and others wake up frequently drenched in sweat. While some women experience sweats during the day, sweating may be more noticeable during the night.

Night sweats, like many of the symptoms of peri-menopause and postmenopause, may be a sign of an illness or condition unrelated to hormones.

Some of the sleep changes that you will experience during the menopausal transition are related to normal aging. The physiologic changes from aging can cause frequent periods of lighter sleep and reduce the time spent in deep sleep. As women age, the amount of needed sleep decreases—from 8 hours or more, to 5 to 7 hours.

Life events have a profound effect on sleep. Many life events, such as the ill health or death of a parent, spouse, or friend; the loss of a job; or an "empty nest" can coincide with the time period of the menopausal transition.

Stress can interfere with quality of sleep. Stress has also been known to increase menopausal symptoms. As menopausal symptoms get worse, you can become more stressed and less able to sleep. Less sleep causes fatigue, irritability, and a decreased ability to cope with stress, again interfering with sleep. This causes a cycle of too much stress and too little sleep.

Inability to sleep can be frustrating at the time, but it can also be a real problem the next day and over time. Sleep loss has been linked with poor concentration, reasoning, and remembering; poor functioning at school or work; fatigue; mood changes; depression; and headache. Most of these symptoms have also been linked to menopause.

Heather's comment:

Sleep, I used to sleep so well. Just like a baby. Not now, now I'm asleep, then I wake up hot and sopping wet. Then

I am freezing while I am up changing the bed. I have to keep extra sheets and tee shirts beside the bed, and every morning I take them all down to the washer and wash them, and take them back up stairs at night—it is ridiculous. Sometimes I just laugh...

Bridget's comment:

It was sleep-disturbed nights that finally got to me, though. Every hour or two, I'd thrash around and throw off the covers. Nighttime hot flashes offered an additional feature: an uncontrollable urge to empty my bladder, full or not. Several times a night, I'd wake up drenched in sweat and shuffle into the bathroom. For a while I was sure I had diabetes. After a few months, I couldn't stand it anymore. I gave in and started taking estrogen and progesterone. Every symptom disappeared in no time. A year later, I tried to stop hormone therapy. The sweating and sleep disturbances returned within two weeks, and I was back at the prescription counter in a flash. No pun intended.

32. Why do I get symptoms one day and not the next?

You are not imagining that your symptoms change from day to day. Sometimes the change in symptoms is a direct result of changes in levels of hormones, and sometimes it's how well you cope when you haven't slept well, or when you're overwhelmed with work or family concerns.

There is a physical reason for your symptoms, but how you respond to them will probably vary from day to day based on how much sleep you're getting or what's on your mind. If you're feeling irritable, your hot flashes are probably going to feel much worse.

"Hormonal chaos" can make your symptoms worse one day and disappear the next. This is particularly true for hot flashes. As hormone levels change abruptly during perimenopause, hot flashes will occur more frequently, and as hormone levels start to even off after menopause, symptoms like hot flashes will eventually occur less frequently and become less intense.

33. I'm not on any hormone therapy and have not had a menstrual period for 5 years. I started bleeding again several days ago. Is that normal?

Bleeding in postmenopause is never normal.

No. Bleeding in postmenopause is never normal. You should contact your clinician as soon as possible if you experience either spotting or bleeding once your periods have stopped for a full year. Sometimes women will ignore bleeding after intercourse, thinking that it's just caused by vaginal dryness. But it can't be overemphasized: Bleeding is abnormal in postmenopause until proven otherwise.

Infections can cause bleeding, and sometimes clinicians will want to wait until bleeding stops so that the cultures taken to test for infection can be interpreted more easily by the laboratory. The vaginal dryness from low estrogen can cause the vaginal walls and cervix to bleed.

If you are on estrogen-progestin therapy, you may get a regular period and some breakthrough bleeding in the early months of being on the therapy. If you have not been bleeding on the HT that you are taking and bleeding occurs, contact your clinician to discuss it.

Some **over-the-counter (OTC)** products, including **black cohosh,** may cause bleeding when you stop taking them. That's why it's so important that you tell your clinician if you're taking any OTC products.

Although abnormal cells and cancer cells in the cervix, vaginal wall, and endometrium can also cause bleeding, your spotting could be a fluke. However, spotting or bleeding must be taken seriously until you have discussed it with your clinician. You can expect that your clinician will take a history of any other symptoms that may accompany the bleeding or spotting, such as bloating, abdominal or back pain, fever, and weight gain or loss. You can also expect that your clinician will examine you, take cultures, and do a pregnancy test if necessary. S/he may also take an endometrial biopsy, which involves inserting an instrument through the cervix and taking a small piece of tissue to send to a pathology lab. Your clinician may order a vaginal ultrasound, which allows the uterus, ovaries, and fallopian tubes to be examined more completely by viewing them through the vaginal wall.

Other causes of abnormal bleeding include bleeding disorders, thyroid disease, pituitary gland tumors, or fibroids or polyps in the cervix or uterus.

Gayle's comment:

I hadn't had a period in 3 years. And one day, I just started bleeding. How could this be? I bled for a week before I finally called my doctor. He didn't want to see me until the bleeding stopped, which it did in another several days. I was really worried that I would need a hysterectomy. My doctor wanted me to have a procedure where he could see

Over-the-counter (OTC)

describes medications, herbs, or supplements that can be bought without a prescription.

Black cohosh

an herb in the buttercup family used frequently in Native American medicine for a variety of ailments, including rheumatism, colds, constipation, backache and gynecological disorders. Also called black snakeroot, bugwort, bugbane, rattleroot, rattletop, macrotys, and squawroot. Used by many women to treat hot flashes.

*inside the uterus, take a tissue sample, and then do a D &
C. The procedure was a breeze. Of course I was asleep the
whole time! I had to wait several weeks for the results, but
his first impression was right—there was nothing wrong.
It was just one of those strange things that can happen
with hormones! I was so relieved.*

PART THREE

Evaluating Symptoms: Is It Menopause?

Are there health problems that should I be screened for as I approach menopause and after?

What is osteoporosis? I've heard that I'm at greater risk for it during menopause. Is that true? Why am I more at risk for osteoporosis during postmenopause?

How do I know if I'm depressed?

Am I more likely to get breast, endometrial, ovarian, or cervical cancer after menopause?

More ...

34. How will having a longer menstrual life and later menopause affect my health?

Because women have an increased number of menstrual cycles overall than in the past (see Question 11 discussing menstrual life), they also have a slightly increased risk of certain cancers and other health conditions. Every ovulation increases hormone levels, so women who have a longer menstrual life will have some increased risk for hormone-linked cancers, like cancer of the ovary, breast, or lining of the uterus (see Question 43 discussing risks for certain cancers). But having more periods has some benefits, too. The higher levels of estrogen help increase bone strength and lower the risk of later getting osteoporosis (see Question 37 discussing osteoporosis).

Some experts say that a shorter menstrual life, shortened by pregnancy and breastfeeding, starting periods later, or having menopause earlier, helps reduce the risk of getting ovarian, breast, and uterine cancers. Breastfeeding and pregnancy help to decrease the risk partly because the menstrual cycle is interrupted, and hormone fluctuations are reduced. This is why some women's health experts suggest using birth control pills or patches, because using hormones for birth control puts the body into a state more like the ancient hunter/gatherer societies when women had fewer menstrual cycles due to the fact that they were usually pregnant or breastfeeding. Fewer cycles can decrease the risk of some cancers.

PMS (premenstrual syndrome) is a bigger problem for women today because we have more menstrual cycles.

Premenstrual dysphoric disorder (PMDD) is a more serious problem when women have depression before and during their periods. PMS may develop for the first time or become worse during perimenopause. More periods can mean more pain for those with endometriosis. Although the cause is not really known, one theory about endometriosis is that it is caused when menstrual blood and tissue goes out of the fallopian tubes, and attaches to organs and tissues in the belly. During menstruation, severe pain can be experienced in all of the areas where the tissue has attached. More periods can also increase the chance for anemia (low red blood cell count) in women who experience extremely heavy periods because of the blood loss with more menstrual cycles.

35. Are there health problems that I should be screened for as I approach menopause and after?

Menopause is a totally normal and natural process. But many of the symptoms that you can experience during perimenopause and after can also be due to health problems that are often experienced at midlife, such as diabetes and thyroid disease, high blood pressure, abnormal heart rhythms, chest pain, low blood counts, depression, anxiety, infections, or cancer. Irregular bleeding, particularly after menopause, should always be checked by your clinician because it might be a sign of pregnancy, fibroids, cancer, or other problems in the uterus.

Menopause is a totally normal and natural process.

Sometimes a woman's perimenopausal symptoms are better when medical problems are treated. For example, you may go to your clinician for vague symptoms like fatigue and headache, thinking that these symptoms are due to menopause. You may find out that you have high blood pressure, diabetes, or thyroid disease. After the real problem is treated, your fatigue and headaches related to menopause may disappear or at least be less annoying.

So, although perimenopause and menopause are natural processes that occur at midlife, it's important to be screened for health problems that can also occur at midlife. See Table 3 for screening tests that you might want to have. Having a complete physical every year or two after menopause is usually often enough, but you may need to be checked more often if you have chronic diseases, or are having health problems or concerns.

It's important to be screened for health problems that can also occur at midlife.

36. I understand that being overweight as well as menopausal puts me at risk for a number of health problems. It's not that easy to lose weight. Does it really matter?

Yes, it does matter. A lot. Almost two thirds of Americans are overweight, and obesity is the second leading cause of death in the United States. **Body Mass Index** (BMI) is used as a way to tell exactly how overweight you are. Both your height and weight are used to calculate your BMI (see Figure 9 for the calculation). You can have your BMI calculated for you on the Internet at *www.obesity.org* (American Obesity Association), and at the Web site for the Centers for Disease Control and Prevention *www.cdc.gov/nccdphp/dnpa/bmi/calc-bmi.htm*. If your BMI is between 18 and 25, you are in the healthy range. If your BMI is between 25 and 30, you are overweight. If your BMI is over 30, you are obese. If a woman is 5 feet 6 inches tall and

Body Mass Index (BMI)

a measurement of body size that includes both height and weight. It is calculated by dividing your weight (in pounds) by your height (in inches) squared, multiplied by 704.5.

Table 3   Midlife Health Screening

Health Concern	Screening Method	Frequency*
Bladder disease	Urinalysis	Yearly after 50**
Breast cancer	Breast self-exam (BSE)	
	Breast exam by clinician	Monthly **
		Yearly
	Mammogram	Every 1 to 2 years starting at age 40; then yearly starting at age 50
Cervical cancer	Pap smear	Every 2 to 3 years (if no prior abnormal)
Colon cancer	Sigmoidoscopy OR	Every 5 years, starting at age 50, with yearly testing for blood in the stool
	Colonoscopy OR	Every 10 years starting at age 50
	Barium enema	Every 5 to 10 years starting at age 50
Dental disease	Dental exam	Every 6 months or yearly
Diabetes	Fasting blood sugar	Every 3 years starting at age 45
Eye disease/vision	Eye examination	Every 2-4 years starting at age 40
		Every 1 to 2 years starting at age 65
Heart Disease	Blood pressure measurement	Yearly
	Fasting blood cholesterol panel	Every 5 years starting at age 45
	ECG or EKG (electrocardiogram)	At age 40**
Osteoporosis/Osteopenia	Height measurement	Yearly
	Bone density measurement	Age 65
Overweight/obesity	Height and weight measurement	Yearly
	Waist measurement	Yearly‡
Skin cancer	Self-exam	Monthly
	Exam by clinician	Yearly
Thyroid disease	Thyroid stimulating hormone level	Every 5 years starting at age 35**

*Frequency recommendations are based on the average risk person; more frequent screening or additional screening tests may be needed for women with high risk due to personal or family history, or who are experiencing symptoms.

**Controversial

‡To identify excessive abdominal fat tissue, not done by all clinicians, which can be measured at home.

$$\frac{\text{Weight in pounds}}{(\text{Height in inches})^2} \times 704.5 = BMI$$

Figure 9   Calculating your Body Mass Index (BMI).

weighs 164 pounds, her BMI is 26.4. She is over-weight. If she lost just 10 pounds and weighed 154, her BMI would be in the normal range at 24.9.

In the United States, more people are overweight than underweight. But being underweight is not healthy either. And midlife women are not immune to eating disorders like **anorexia nervosa** or **bulimia**. The **binge eating disorder**, when a person eats very large amounts of food at a single sitting, is also more common among midlife women than you might imagine. So, if you are underweight (have a BMI of less than 18), overweight (BMI over 25), or have an eating disorder, you should seek evaluation and guidance about how to regain a normal BMI in a healthy way.

Having a BMI over 27 has been associated with having a higher frequency of menopause symptoms such as night sweats, hot flashes, and neck, back, or shoulder soreness or stiffness. Obesity also puts you at risk for a number of health-related problems, such as:

* high blood pressure
* high blood cholesterol
* diabetes
* hardening or blockage of the arteries
* stroke
* heart failure
* gallstones
* gout (painful and swollen joints)

Anorexia nervosa

a disorder characterized by fear of becoming obese, thinking the body is larger than it really is, severe weight loss, and an aversion to food. Once thought to only affect teenage girls, it is now recognized in women of all ages.

Bulimia

an eating disorder that usually includes episodes of binge eating (eating very large amounts of food) and purging (forcing vomiting or diarrhea to get food out of the system).

Binge eating disorder

a disorder characterized by eating very large quantities of food in short periods of time, usually leads to being overweight or obese.

- arthritis
- sleep disturbances
- some types of cancer (colon, breast, or the lining of the uterus)
- problems with pregnancy
- menstrual irregularities, infertility
- urine incontinence
- kidney stones

The diabetes that you develop as an adult is called Type 2 diabetes and is much more common as you age. Your changing hormones will not increase your risk of diabetes, but if you have diabetes, your shifting hormone levels can make it more difficult to keep your diabetes under control. Diabetes affects women of color more than white women.

There are some risks for getting Type 2 diabetes. Some of them you can control, others you can't:

- BMI over 25
- A waist measure of more than 35 inches (you can have a "healthy" BMI but still be at risk if you have a lot of fat tissue around your middle)
- An inactive lifestyle
- Having diabetes when pregnant
- A family history of diabetes
- High blood pressure
- High blood **lipids**
- **Insulin resistance** (high levels of insulin or difficulty with the body using insulin)
- Polycystic ovary syndrome (a syndrome of being overweight, having irregular menstrual patterns, difficulty with the body using insulin, extra hair growth, acne, and possibly multiple cysts in the ovaries)

If you have diabetes, your shifting hormone levels can make it more difficult to keep your diabetes under control.

Lipids

generally considered to be the fats and cholesterol found in blood. Higher density lipids are the "good" fats, and the lower density lipids are the "bad" fats.

Insulin resistance

insulin has difficulty carrying sugar into body cells (the cells are resistant). High levels of insulin, and sometimes blood sugar, results. People with insulin resistance are at higher risk for developing diabetes.

Screening for diabetes is important around the age of 45, and every 3 years after that if your fasting blood sugar (FBS) is normal (<100 mg/dL). You should be screened at an earlier age if you have any of the risks listed above. If your fasting blood sugar level is slightly high, you might be asked to have some additional testing along with changing your diet and exercise. Besides increasing your risk for heart disease, diabetes also increases your risk for infections, foot ulcers, circulation problems, kidney disease, and blindness.

If you develop or already have diabetes, controlling your blood sugar can be harder during perimenopause because both estrogen and progesterone influence how your body uses insulin and blood sugar. And, symptoms of high or low blood sugar can be mistaken for signs of perimenopause, like having hot flashes or feeling weak or tired. So, if you're overweight and you are having any of these symptoms, you should ask your clinician about getting a fasting blood sugar test for diabetes. If you do have diabetes, getting it under control may reduce your perimenopausal symptoms as well.

It's hard to lose weight and exercise, but if you do, you'll lower your risk for diseases and live a healthier, longer life.

Perimenopause can be a time when you feel that you are losing something, and it's probably not weight! For some women, the upcoming loss of fertility is of great concern. For others, the loss of control and predictability of periods and moodiness can be of even more concern. But what you *can* control is your lifestyle. If you are overweight and don't lose the weight before you get to menopause, you have even more risk of diabetes and heart disease, and you might have more menopausal symptoms. Yes, it's hard to lose weight and exercise, but if you do, you'll lower your risk for diseases and live a healthier, longer life.

37. What is osteoporosis? I've heard that I'm at greater risk for it after menopause. Is that true? Why am I more at risk for osteoporosis during postmenopause?

Osteoporosis is a loss in bone density that makes bone more fragile and easy to break. In adults, bone goes through a normal process where old bone is broken down and new bone is formed all the time. Osteoporosis happens when this process gets out of balance and there is more bone breakdown than there is new bone being formed. It results in weak bone. Osteoporosis and osteopenia are a little bit different. The difference has to do with how much bone is lost. Osteopenia means some bone has been lost, but the risk for breaking bone is not very high. Osteoporosis means that more bone has been lost and the risk for breaking a bone is high.

There is a complex system that helps to maintain the balance between building and breaking down bone. Several hormones, including estrogen, progesterone, androgens, thyroid and growth hormones, steroids, and minerals like calcium and phosphorus contribute to the balance of the bone cycle. Testosterone, in particular, has a positive effect on the cycle, creating greater bone density, which is one reason why men don't get osteoporosis as frequently as women. They start with stronger bones, and lose bone more slowly because their testosterone levels are much higher than in women.

It's absolutely true that you are at higher risk for osteoporosis after menopause.

Yes, it's absolutely true that you are at higher risk for osteoporosis after menopause. And the reason is that estrogen has a big effect on bone. Once the estrogen levels decrease following menopause, the rate of bone loss goes up and passes the rate of new bone being formed. The bone loss that postmenopausal women have is more rapid and more severe, especially in the first 5 to 7 years after menopause. In fact, about one fifth of a woman's total bone loss will happen in those first 5 to 7 years. The density of the bone decreases over time, making the bone more susceptible to fractures. Overall, more women than men have osteoporosis, and more women have broken bones as a result.

Osteopenia and osteoporosis are not painful, unless, of course, you break a bone or your spine starts to deteriorate. It does not give you symptoms. You won't even know that you have it unless you are tested for it or you break a bone. The other way it may be detected is by the "dowager's hump" (kyphosis), a hunched-back appearance (see Figure 10) that happens when the front edges of the bones of the spine collapse from tiny breaks, causing the spine to bend forward.

The "dowager's hump" causes other problems over time. As the "hunch" becomes worse, organs get compressed, causing pain, indigestion, acid reflux from the stomach, incontinence, constipation, difficulty breathing, mobility problems, and fatigue. A woman's height decreases over time as the spine bends forward. This is not normal and indicates bone loss. Your clinician should be measuring your height at annual visits, particularly when you reach menopause, to detect any small changes in height.

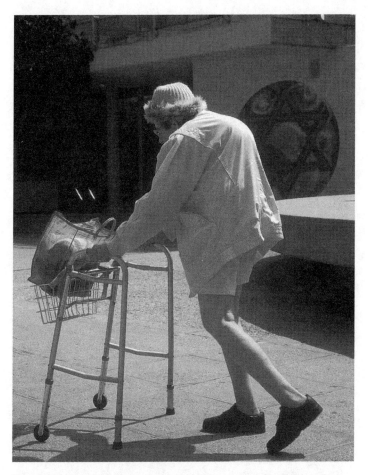

Figure 10 Dowager's hump. In people with osteoporosis, the bones in the upper spine develop small compression fractures. These bones heal into wedge shapes, and the upper spine assumes a deformed, curved shape known as "dowager's hump."

The main problem associated with osteoporosis is the risk of breaking a bone, and the toll on women following broken bones can be very high. About half of all women who have a broken hip will have some form of permanent disability. Almost one in four will die in the first year after the break. Of those who live, about 20% will be sent to long-term nursing home care. The cost from broken hips is both financial and social. Healthcare costs are high, there is increased risk for death and disability, and many women won't be able to return to their normal activities. This makes osteoporosis a huge problem and a huge risk for you as you enter menopause, even though you can't see it and you can't feel it.

38. When should I be tested for osteoporosis? How is osteoporosis diagnosed?

The National Osteoporosis Foundation (NOF) recommends testing in women who are postmenopausal and at least 65 years of age, or in younger women who have risks for bone loss besides age, gender, or race (see risks below). The NOF also recommends testing for all women who are 65 or older regardless of risks, for postmenopausal women who have had a broken bone, and for women who are considering medications and therapies to treat osteoporosis to help them make more informed decisions (Figure 11).

According to the National Osteoporosis Foundation, the following risk factors for osteoporosis should be assessed when testing is being considered:

- *Age*: As you get older, you are more likely to develop osteoporosis.
- *Gender*: Females far outnumber males with osteoporosis.
- *Lifestyle factors*: Low intake of calcium and Vitamin D, limited exercise, cigarette smoking, and excessive

What should I do about osteoporosis?

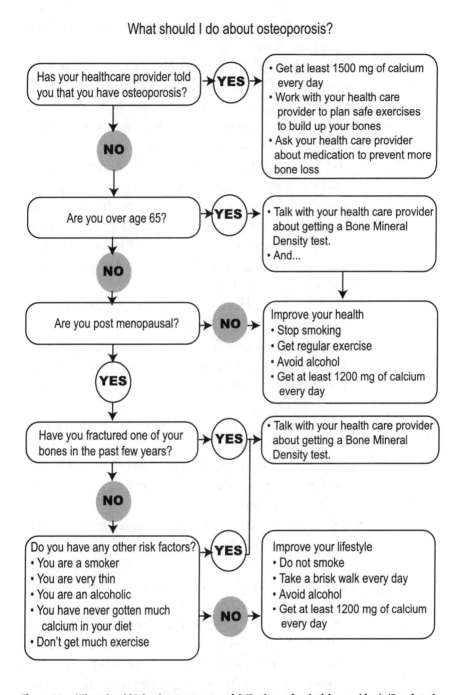

Figure 11   What should I do about osteoporosis? (Pathway for decision making). (Reprinted with permission from *Journal of Midwifery and Women's Health* Vol. 48-1, p. 72, "Share with women".)

use of caffeine, soda beverages, or alcohol can contribute to bone loss.

- *Low body weight*: If you weigh less than 127 pounds and are small-boned, or have a BMI of less than 20, you are at higher risk for bone loss (see Question 36 about BMI). Estrogen levels are generally higher in overweight or obese women because the fat tissue converts androgens to estrogen. The extra estrogen provides some protection against bone loss. Heavier women also tend to develop greater bone strength due to the extra weight the bones support. Fat tissue in heavier women may also provide some protection against breaking bones from a fall because it provides some natural padding.

- *Family history*: If your mother or grandmother has osteoporosis you are also at greater risk.

- *Race*: Caucasian or Asian women are at higher risk than African-American or Hispanic women. But osteoporosis is still an important problem for Hispanic and African-American women.

- *Menopause history*: Premature menopause or menopause induced by surgery, chemotherapy, or radiation may increase your risk for bone loss because of the sudden and extended period of time without estrogen.

- *Medications*: There are many medications that can increase the risk for bone loss, such as those used to treat intestinal disorders, seizure disorders, blood clotting disorders, endometriosis, rheumatoid arthritis, asthma, and cancer. Long-term use of steroids, such as prednisone, can have a particularly bad effect on bones, as can some illnesses, such as overproduction of thyroid hormone (hyperthyroidism) or overproduction of steroids (Cushing's disease).

There are several tests that are used to evaluate bone density so that your clinician can diagnose osteoporosis and osteopenia. All are painless, safe, and not invasive. See Figure 12, which demonstrates how bone density testing is easy and not invasive.

If your clinician sends you for a DEXA/DXA (dual energy x-ray absorptiometry), you can expect to have your hip, spine, or whole body evaluated. The test takes about 5 minutes. This is the "gold standard" or the top test for diagnosing both osteoporosis and osteopenia. Testing can also be done on outer limbs such as wrists, heels, or lower arms. These tests are only good for screening because the diagnosis of osteoporosis is only made when central bones such as the hip or spine are evaluated. So, if your screening test shows low bone density, it is likely that your clinician would advise a test for your hip or spine.

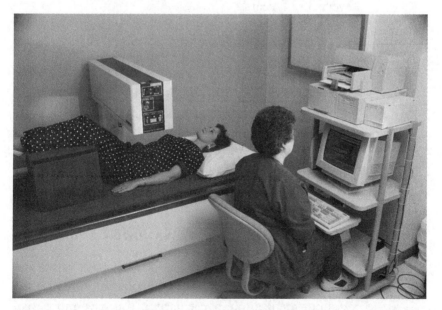

Figure 12   Bone mineral density tests are painless, noninvasive, and safe; bone density may be measured in the spine, hip, wrist, finger, kneecap, shin bone, or heel, depending on the machine.

Bone density testing should be avoided during pregnancy, immediately after other x-ray studies that were done with contrast dye, or if the person weighs more than 250 pounds (because most DXA machines cannot accommodate individuals of that size). You should not take calcium supplements in the 24 hours before your test. Wear comfortable and loose clothing without metal clasps. Avoid wearing an underwire bra or a navel ring.

Once you are diagnosed with osteoporosis, you will be tested at intervals to check the effects of treatments and to see if there are any changes over time. Your spine will show the changes most quickly, but most clinicians follow measurements at both the hip and spine. You can expect to have repeat tests every 1 to 2 years at first. Once you have two tests in a row that show similar results, then testing may only be needed every 3 to 5 years.

Jackie's comment:

Because I had an early menopause, I had my first bone density test in my early 40s. My BMD was a little abnormal in my hips. My doctor told me to just start walking. Now I'm adding the resistance training. I sit here with my 5-pound weights. When I walk, I really pump my arms. Here in Florida, I can walk every day without worrying about the cold weather. I walk about 8–10 miles per week.

39. Can I prevent osteoporosis from happening to me?

You may not be able to totally prevent osteoporosis without medication, particularly if you have more than one risk (see Question 37 on who should be tested). But you can do the following things to decrease bone loss:

- You can increase your intake of calcium, Vitamin D, and magnesium to improve the strength of your bones. The National Academy of Sciences recommends that women over 51 years of age get 1,300 mg of **elemental calcium** each day. The National Institutes of Health suggests 1,500 mg/day, so getting between 1,300 mg and 1,500 mg is probably a good idea. Perimenopausal women who are not pregnant or breastfeeding need less elemental calcium, and 1,000 mg/day is recommended. Elemental calcium refers to the calcium that your body can absorb and use. If you are not getting enough calcium in your diet, you should be taking a calcium supplement (see Table 4 for the different types of calcium, Table 5 for food sources of calcium, and Question 40 about calcium supplements). The daily requirement for Vitamin D is 400-800 IU (international units). Vitamin D is found in fatty fish, fortified milk, and daily vitamin supplements, and can

Elemental calcium
the calcium that your body absorbs and uses.

Table 4   Calcium Supplements

Type of Calcium	Amount of Elemental Calcium	Amount of Elemental Calcium Absorbed per 1,000 mg	Sample Product Names
Calcium Carbonate*	40.0%	400 mg	Various, e.g., Tums, Oscal
Calcium Citrate*	21.1%	211 mg	Citracal
Calcium Glubionate	6.4%	64 mg	Neo-glucagon syrup
Calcium Gluconate	9.0%	90 mg	Various
Calcium Phosphate Tribasic	37.5%	375 mg	Posture

*Most frequently used supplements

Table 5 Food Sources of Calcium

Food Source	Serving Size	Calcium Amount
Tofu (with calcium sulfate)	½ cup	434 mg
Milk, Skim	1 cup	321 mg
Yogurt, Low Fat	1 cup	300 mg
Calcium Fortified Orange Juice	8 oz	300 mg
Milk, Whole	1 cup	291 mg
Milk, Whole, Chocolate	1 cup	280 mg
Swiss Cheese	1 slice	270 mg
Collard greens (cooked)	1 cup	226 mg
Monterey Jack Cheese	1 slice	210 mg
Canned Sardines (with bones)*	3 oz	204 mg
Cheddar Cheese	1 slice	200 mg
Canned Salmon (with bones)*	3 oz	181 mg
Broccoli	1 cup	180 mg
American Cheese	1 slice	174 mg
Mozzarella Cheese	1 slice	174 mg
Yogurt, Frozen	½ cup	152 mg
Bread (calcium fortified)	1 slice	150 mg
Turnip greens (cooked)	1 cup	147 mg
Cottage Cheese	1 cup	140 mg
Mustard Greens	1 cup	103 mg
Almonds	½ cup	92 mg
Ice Cream	½ cup	75 mg
Cereal (calcium fortified)	1 cup	Varies

Spinach and Swiss chard have binders that can interfere with calcium absorption.
*Calcium content includes eating the bones.

be absorbed through the skin with sunlight exposure. Vitamin D is needed for your body to absorb calcium. The RDA for magnesium is 320 mg from food sources. Food sources of magnesium include spinach, broccoli, beans, cashews, sunflower seeds, halibut, whole wheat bread, and milk.

- Stop smoking cigarettes. Cigarette smokers have an earlier menopause, which in itself puts you at higher risk for bone loss. Smokers also have more broken bones than nonsmokers, partly because nicotine increases bone loss by interfering with the process of bone development.

- Limit alcohol, soda beverages, and caffeine intake. These products interfere with the process of bone development, and contribute to bone loss.

- Avoid medications that can decrease bone mass, including some anticonvulsants or injectable blood thinners (heparin). Sometimes your clinician will be able to find different medications that are less damaging to bone, and some medications may be taken in shorter courses, such as steroids.

- Exercise regularly and do strength training with weights as part of your routine. People generally understand how exercise makes your muscles stronger. But why exercise is so important to keeping your bones healthy is a little less clear. Bone, because it is a live tissue and is constantly developing, will actually strengthen if given the right amount of stress. Stress in this sense means carrying weight and pushing against weight. In other words, exercise! To increase your bone strength, do weight-bearing exercises like brisk walking, jogging or cycling, as well as strength-training exercises like lifting weights or push-ups. Lifting even 5 or 10 pounds will make a huge difference in wrist strength. Over time, weight-bearing exercise and strength training will increase bone mass, improve muscle strength, and also improve your balance so you are less likely to fall in the first place. See Table 6 for tips on preventing falls. Exercise works where

Table 6   Tips to Prevent Falls

Outdoors

- Use a cane or walker for added stability.
- Wear rubber-soled shoes for traction.
- Walk on grass when sidewalks are slippery.
- In winter, carry salt to sprinkle on slippery sidewalks.

Indoors

- Keep rooms free of clutter, especially on the floors.
- Be careful on highly polished floors that become slick and dangerous when wet.
- Avoid walking in socks, stockings, or slippers without rubber soles.
- Be sure carpets and area rugs have skid-proof backing or are tacked to the floor.
- Keep stairwells well lit.
- Attach handrails on both sides of all stairwells.
- Install grab bars on bathroom walls near tub, shower, and toilet.
- Use a rubber bath mat in shower or tub.
- Keep a flashlight with fresh batteries beside the bed.

Bone strength will benefit in the areas where you exercise.

you do it. In other words, bone strength will benefit in the areas where you exercise—walking benefits the leg, hip, and lower spine bones; lifting weights helps the arm, wrist, and upper spine bones. Some exercises should be avoided if you have bone loss already, mainly those that require bending forward at the waist. Forward bending can increase the stress on the front of the spine bones too much, and instead of strengthening bone can actually cause tiny breaks (see Question 37 about osteoporosis and the "dowager's hump"). Instead, do exercises that involve arching your back, or modify toe touching and forward bending movements so your spine remains straight.

- You can take medications to help reduce bone loss (see Table 7 for treatment options).

Madeline's comment:

I just had a bone density test and my bones are perfect. I worried because I went through menopause so young—13 years ago. I'm good about taking calcium supplements. I laugh a little about needing to do regular exercise because I have a paper route and the newspaper bundles can be quite heavy. Sometimes the Sunday paper can weigh as much as 5 pounds, and by putting those papers into the mail tubes, I get my resistance training in! I think that must be helping my bones. I know I should do more exercise than just being as active as I am. I'm on my feet all day being a hair stylist and shop owner, so it's hard to think about walking too, but I know I should. When I deliver the newspapers, I take little "power walks" in between. I'm diabetic too, I have high blood pressure, I'm hypothyroid, a little overweight but at least my bones are in good shape!

40. Is there any treatment for osteoporosis?

Osteoporosis is usually treated with exercise, assuring you are getting enough calcium and Vitamin D, and medication that most suits your level of bone loss. You also need to think about other illnesses you may have that can interfere with the medication, what medication side effects you can tolerate, and whether you have other symptoms that might benefit from one treatment over another. See Table 7 for management options for osteopenia and osteoporosis.

If you are diagnosed with osteopenia or osteoporosis, it is critical that you take calcium supplements to help

Table 7 Medications and Supplements for Osteopenia and Osteoporosis in Postmenopausal Women

Medication or Supplements	Clinical Uses in Post-menopausal Bone Loss	Considerations
Alendronate (Fosamax)	Osteopenia & Osteoporosis	• Take first thing in the morning on an empty stomach with a full glass of water, remain upright, and take no other food or drink for at least 30 minutes • Can be taken once per week • Take 2 hours before antacids/calcium • Caution if allergic; upper gastrointestinal disease, e.g., ulcers or reflux; or kidney disease • May cause inflammation of stomach or esophagus, nausea, vomiting, constipation, diarrhea, flatulence, ulcer, swelling, or abdominal, muscle, back, or joint pain
Calcitonin (Miacalcin)	Osteoporosis	• Usually administered as a nasal spray • Has pain relieving effect on fractures due to osteoporosis • Caution if allergic • May cause spasms of large airways, nausea, vomiting, flushing, rash, itching, warmth, nighttime urination, eye pain, reduced appetite, swelling, abdominal pain, salty taste, or Paget's disease (thickening and softening of bone)
Calcium (Tums, Viactiv, Citracal, OsCal, Posture, fortified orange juice, others)	Osteopenia & Osteoporosis Prevention Needed even if normal bone strength, or if taking other medications for bone loss	• 1,300 to 1,500 mg of elemental calcium should be taken daily • Depending on type of calcium supplement (see Table 4 Calcium Supplements), varying amounts of calcium absorbed • Change type of calcium if you get stomach upset, gas, constipation • Not absorbed well when taken with leafy greens, caffeine, iron, or excessive salt • Calcium and magnesium taken together may reduce hot flashes, as well • Available over-the-counter

Table 7   (continued)

Medication or Supplements	Clinical Uses in Post-menopausal Bone Loss	Considerations
Estrogen (e.g., Activella*, Alora , Climara, Estrace, Estraderm, Estratab, Femhrt*, Menest, Menostar±, Ortho-prefest*, Premarin, Vivelle, Vivelle Dot, others)	Osteopenia & Osteoporosis	• Also effective in alleviating most symptoms of menopause • Improves balance and reduces falls • Comes in several forms (i.e., pills, patch, ring, cream, gel) • ±Menostar: very low dose estrogen patch specifically tested and prescribed for reducing risk of osteoporosis, may not provide relief of hot flashes since dose is so low • See Appendix B, table of commonly used hormone therapies
Isoflavones (Promensil, Rimostil, others)	May help to prevent osteopenia and osteoporosis	• Isoflavones derived from red clover • May also help reduce hot flashes • Long-term safety not yet determined • Can be taken with other prescribed medications to treat osteoporosis • Available over-the-counter
Raloxifene (Evista)	Osteopenia & Osteoporosis	• Not recommended if taking ET or EPT • Caution if allergy, blood clots, high triglyceride levels, using hormone therapy • May cause hot flashes, infection, flu-like symptoms, joint pain, sinusitis, nausea, weight gain, inflammation of mouth/throat, depression, cough, leg cramps, rash, insomnia, stomach upset, or clots
Risedronate (Actonel)	Osteopenia & Osteoporosis	• Take first thing in the morning on an empty stomach with a full glass of water, remain upright, and take no other food or drink for at least 30 minutes • Can be taken once per week • Take 2 hours before antacids/calcium • Caution if allergic; upper gastrointestinal disease, e.g., ulcers or reflux; or kidney disease

Table 7 (continued)

Medication or Supplements	Clinical Uses in Post menopausal Bone Loss	Considerations
Risedronate (Actonel) (continued)	Osteopenia & Osteoporosis	• May cause inflammation of stomach or esophagus, nausea, vomiting, constipation, diarrhea, flatulence, ulcer, swelling, or abdominal, muscle, back, or joint pain
Teriparitide (Forteo)	Osteoporosis	• Given by injection • Usually used only if other treatments are ineffective • Caution if allergy, bone cancer, history of radiation to bone, urinary stones, parathyroid disease, bone disease • May cause low blood pressure, dizziness, weakness, joint pain, leg cramps, fainting, chest pain
Vitamins, minerals (Vitamin D, B Vitamins, Folate, magnesium, phosphorus)	All have role in maintaining bone health, and some may help to prevent osteoporosis and fractures associated with it	• May be taken as a vitamin supplement or taken separately • Vitamin B and folate help to lower high homocysteine levels associated with osteoporosis and fractures • Vitamin D improves balance and reduces falls • Can be taken with any prescribed treatment for osteoporosis • Available over-the-counter

*Also contain progesterone compounds.

**All medications have associated benefits, risks, and side effects; we have listed only those that may be especially pertinent for postmenopausal women. See the section discussing hormone therapy for more information regarding estrogen and progestins.

Homocysteine

an amino acid that is being studied for its role in increasing heart disease and osteoporosis. Vitamin B and folate are known to reduce homocysteine levels.

slow the progression of bone loss. Even if you have not been diagnosed with either one, it is still important for you to get enough calcium in your diet or to take calcium supplements daily. Taking Vitamin B and folate (folic acid) will also help by reducing **homocysteine** levels. High levels of homocysteine may weaken your bones, making them more likely to break.

Calcium comes in several forms. Regardless of the type of calcium, it's most important that your calcium intake meets or exceeds 1,300–1,500 mg per day of elemental calcium if you are postmenopausal and not using hormone therapy. Although you might think that you are getting enough calcium from your supplements, only a certain percentage of the calcium supplement you are taking is usable as elemental calcium. Elemental calcium is what your body can actually absorb and use. See Table 4 (page 79) describing the different forms of calcium, and how much elemental calcium is contained in each variety. It's also important to get enough Vitamin D so that calcium can be absorbed through the intestines. The following forms of calcium are available and contain the most elemental calcium (the amount that your system can absorb):

- *Calcium carbonate.* Calcium carbonate is best taken at meals because it is best absorbed in an acidic environment. It comes in chewable tablets, tablets you swallow whole, and liquid. Taking preparations that also have magnesium can reduce the gas and constipation that often comes with calcium carbonate. Examples of calcium carbonate include Tums®, Rolaids®, Viactiv®, Os-Cal®, and Mylanta®. Questions have been raised recently about the use of crushed bone meal and oyster shells to make calcium carbonate, and the possibility of lead or arsenic contamination. If there were any contamination, the amount of lead or arsenic would be very small and not likely harmful.
- *Calcium citrate.* This form is absorbed well without acid, so it can be taken at bedtime or on an empty stomach, and is a better choice if you have stomach problems and need to take antacids or acid blockers

(Tums® are used as antacids, so you may be getting calcium in your antacids, too). Citracal® is an example of calcium citrate.

- *Calcium phosphate.* This type of calcium is most often found in fortified beverages like orange juice, or by itself in a product called Posture®.
- *Calcium gluconate* and *calcium glubionate.* Both have relatively low levels of absorbable elemental calcium. They are less commonly used.

Some substances and foods can interfere with the absorption of calcium. Too much fiber in your diet slows the rate of calcium absorption, as do high levels of protein. The best time to take calcium is prior to meals or at bedtime. But remember that calcium carbonate is best when your stomach is producing extra acid, like at mealtime.

Isoflavones like **soy** and red clover may also provide some protection against bone loss. A recent study of women who took Rimostil™ (57 mg of isoflavones from red clover) for 6 months had an increase in bone mineral density. See Part 4 for more information on isoflavones and healthy diet choices.

Isoflavones

a type of phytoestrogen found most notably in soy and red clover.

Soy

the substance derived from soybeans, a protein-rich, low-fat legume.

Jackie's comment:

I don't want to take hormones but I do have some bone changes typical of osteoporosis. I guess that's pretty common for someone who went through menopause so early. I'm taking Estroven Bone Density (daily supplement of calcium and isoflavones from soy). I just don't want to take hormones and I think I feel better for not taking them. I really don't even think about taking them anymore, unless I get in a group of people who are talking about menopause.

41. How do I know if I'm depressed?

Women are at higher risk for depression than men. And women who have had depression before are more likely to get depressed again during perimenopause and after. Depression rates are around three times higher in perimenopausal women than in younger women. Depression can also be a bigger problem at midlife in response to menopausal symptoms related to hormonal changes and midlife stresses like family or relationship problems, health concerns (both for yourself and for others), and money or job concerns. See Table 8 for potential midlife stressors.

Women who have had depression before are more likely to get depressed again during perimenopause and after.

According to the National Institute of Mental Health, you should seek the help of a mental health professional if you are experiencing any of the following symptoms for over 2 weeks:

- A persistent sad, anxious, or empty mood
- Feeling hopeless or pessimistic
- Feeling guilty, worthless, or helpless
- Loss of interest or pleasure in hobbies or activities that you usually enjoy, including sex
- Prolonged tiredness, lack of energy
- Difficulty concentrating, remembering, and making decisions
- Difficulty falling or staying asleep, early morning awakening or oversleeping
- Appetite or weight loss, overeating and weight gain (stress eating)
- Thinking about death or about killing yourself
- Feeling restless or irritable
- Persistent physical symptoms that do not respond to treatment like headaches or stomach upset

Table 8   Potential Midlife Stressors

Source of Stress	Nature of Stress
Self	Appearance
	• Aging
	• Weight gain
	Career
	• Job expectations
	• Job loss
	Faith/religious issues
	• Finding a religious community
	• Rejection of religious community
	Fertility
	• Done having children but mourn the loss of not having more
	• Never able to have children
	Finances
	• Paying for college education of children
	• Saving for retirement not happening
	• Employment concerns
	Health
	• Diagnosed with chronic illness or one of many diseases that you are more at risk for at midlife
	• Depression
	• Overcoming addictions
	Perimenopause
	• Coping with symptoms
	• Fear of aging
	Relationship
	• With partner, children, parents
	• With friends
	• With co-workers, employer
Partner/spouse	Financial
	• Job loss
	• Inadequate retirement funds
	Health
	• Diagnosed with chronic illness
	• Overcoming addictions
	Sexual issues
	• Lack of sex drive
	• Sexual function problems
	• Birth control issues

Table 8 Potential Midlife Stressors

Source of Stress	Nature of Stress
Children	Health
	• Childhood illness or disabilities
	• Caring for disabled adult child
	Success
	• College, job distress
	Their spouse and/or children
	• Marital problems
	• Older children moving back home
	• Raising young children or grandchildren
Parents/Extended Family	Downsizing, moving from childhood home
	Health of parents
	• Diagnosed with terminal illness
	• Worsening chronic illness
	• Normal aging
	Caregiving requirements
	• Caring for one or both parents
	Health concerns for siblings
	• Chronic problems
	• Midlife health risks
	Financial
	• Long-term care expenses for parents
	• Employment concerns or health costs for siblings
Community	Friends' health
	Political concerns
	Community issues

Treatment options for depression include counseling, psychotherapy, antidepressant medications, and herbal remedies. Some antidepressant medications can be used to treat both hot flashes and depression. A different dosage might be needed to benefit both, so be sure that both your menopause and mental health clinician know what medications you are taking, as well as all of the symptoms that you are having. See Question 87 about using antidepressants for the treatment of hot flashes.

42. What are some of the other midlife events and stressors that can affect how I react to menopause?

Perimenopause and menopause coincide with midlife, and that may mean more stressors. These stressors may include but are certainly not limited to stress about money, health (for yourself or a family member or friend), relationships, work issues, or menopausal symptoms. See Table 8 for a listing of life stressors that you may encounter at midlife.

43. Am I more likely to get cancer, such as breast, ovarian, endometrial, or cervical, after menopause?

The risk of developing breast cancer does increase naturally with age. At age 50, you have a 1 in 30 chance of getting breast cancer. According to the American Cancer Society, 77% of breast cancers are diagnosed after the age of 50. A woman's lifetime risk of getting breast cancer is 1 in 9 if she lives to be 80.

The risk of developing breast cancer does increase naturally with age.

You can't change some risk factors for getting breast cancer, such as your gender, age, race, inherited genes for breast cancer, previous radiation to the chest, or family history of breast cancer. Never having children, or having your first child after 30 can increase your risk slightly, but you can't change that after the fact. You also can't change when you started or stopped having periods; getting your first period younger than 12, or experiencing menopause after age 55 may slightly increase your risk of getting breast cancer. Taking birth control pills and breast-feeding are shown to lower the risk for developing breast cancer, probably because they reduce the number of menstrual cycles and hormone shifts you would otherwise experience.

You can reduce your risk for breast cancer *now* by doing the following:

- *Reduce alcohol intake.* Two to five drinks per day increases your risk one and a half times over that of a woman who does not drink alcohol at all. One drink per day doesn't seem to have a significant effect on breast cancer risk.
- *Lose weight if you are overweight.* Obesity increases your risk of breast cancer.
- *Increase fiber and reduce fat in your diet.* A diet high in fat may also be related to an increase risk for breast cancer.

Using hormone therapy for menopause symptoms is less risky than being obese. Short-term use, for 5 years or less, has not been shown to increase the risk beyond that of age. After 5 years the risk is slightly increased (less than 1%) for an individual woman. And don't worry about using deodorants or antiperspirants—rumors have circulated for years that they're linked to breast cancer. They're not.

While recent studies have shown that doing breast self-exams has not reduced breast cancer deaths, breast self-exams are still recommended so that women can monitor their own breast health. Once you reach menopause, it's easy to forget to do self-exams, so it's a good idea to pick a monthly event that will remind you to do it (first day of the month, the day you write bills, etc.). Some clinicians recommend doing self-exams in the morning so that if you find a lump, you don't have to spend a sleepless night worrying about making an appointment. Others advise against doing it on Fridays

Breast self-exams are still recommended so that women can monitor their own breast health.

so that you don't have to spend the weekend being concerned. If you feel uncomfortable doing breast self-exams, you might ask your partner to help you or to do them for you. Be sure to report any unusual lump, thickening of the breast tissue, or nipple discharge to your clinician.

Screening for breast cancer includes breast self-exams, having a breast exam by a clinician once a year, and getting regular mammograms after the age of 40. How often you need to have a mammogram is controversial. Most say you should have your first mammogram at the age of 40, and then another one every 1 to 2 years until you reach the age of 50. After the age of 50, you should have a mammogram every year up to the age of 70 or 75. Lots of women decide to keep having mammograms for screening even after the age of 75. Screening for breast cancer does not yet include MRIs (magnetic resonance imaging), even though they may detect some small cancers earlier. Because MRIs are so expensive, they are usually done only on women who are at very high risk for breast cancer (women who carry a breast cancer gene or who have a strong family history of breast cancer).

The less you ovulate, the lower your risk for ovarian cancer. That's why women who have been on birth control pills are less likely to get ovarian cancer. If you carry one of the breast cancer genes (BRCA 1), if you have a family history of ovarian cancer, or if you have never had children, you are at higher risk.

Because ovarian cancer is so difficult to detect in its early and more treatable stage, many women are afraid of getting it. Comedienne Gilda Radner died from ovarian cancer, and her husband, Gene Wilder, publicized the need for screening and early detection. The problem is that there aren't good screening tools for ovarian cancer. The blood test CA-125 is expensive, and its results are not very reliable in identifying ovarian cancer. All women, whether at high risk or not, should have routine pelvic examinations. If you develop unexplained abdominal bloating or fullness, a pelvic ultrasound may be needed. Routine screening for ovarian cancer is not currently recommended.

Like the risk for ovarian cancer, the risk for endometrial cancer (cancer of the uterine lining) is decreased by the use of birth control pills and by having children. But unlike ovarian cancer, endometrial cancer is highly treatable by removing the uterus. Although you can't control risk factors for endometrial cancer, such as beginning your periods early or stopping them late, or having a family history of a particular form of colon cancer, you can make an effort to control obesity and diabetes, both factors that increase the risk for endometrial cancer. If you are in postmenopause, you should report any spotting, bleeding, abnormal vaginal discharge, pelvic pain, or unexplained weight loss to your clinician. Your clinician will mostly likely do a pelvic exam, and possibly an ultrasound or biopsy. If a biopsy is not adequate to make the diagnosis, you may need to have additional testing. If you still have periods, you should also report spotting between periods, heavy bleeding or prolonged bleeding, or unusual discharge, as well as pelvic pain or weight loss to your clinician.

If you are being treated with estrogen for your menopause symptoms and you have a uterus, it is particularly important that you take progestin with the estrogen to prevent the lining of the uterus from thickening, which can also lead to endometrial cancer.

Many women stop having Pap tests when they get to menopause and stop having periods, which prevents them from being screened adequately for cancer of the cervix (the lower end of the uterus). Cervical cancer can usually be treated easily if it is found early enough. Almost all cervical cancers are related to infection with **human papilloma virus (HPV)**, the virus that causes genital warts. But HPV can go for many years without symptoms, so it's very important to continue your regular pelvic exams with Pap tests. Not all forms of HPV will cause cervical cancer. Treatments are based on the type of HPV infection and your risks for cervical cancer.

Human papilloma virus (HPV)

a virus that is transmitted sexually. Some types of HPV are associated with cancer of the cervix.

It's very important to continue your annual pelvic exams with Pap tests.

Symptoms of cervical cancer can include abnormal bleeding or vaginal discharge. You are also more at risk for cervical cancer if you have had many sexual partners, if you are HIV-positive, if you smoke, or if you started having sexual intercourse at an early age. Condoms reduce your risk of getting cervical cancer by reducing your risk of getting genital warts. And getting an annual Pap test will help your clinician detect cervical cancer at an early stage. Once you have had three normal Pap smears 3 years in a row, your clinician may do them less often, particularly if you practice safer sex (use condoms, have one partner) and don't have any other risk factors.

44. Am I at risk for developing cardiovascular disease (heart disease) after menopause?

Although most women think that breast cancer is the number one cause of death for women, this is not true. Heart disease (also known as cardiovascular disease or

CVD) kills more women every year than the next seven causes of death in women combined. It may come as a surprise to learn that since 1984, more women than men have died from heart disease.

Since 1984, more women than men have died from heart disease.

So, yes, you are more at risk after menopause. You have more than a 50% chance of dying from some type of heart disease after the age of 50. If you are a woman of color, you have an even higher risk of dying from heart disease. Even when you live with heart disease, it can cause long-term problems, not just with your heart, but also with your eyes, kidneys, and other organs.

It has recently been speculated that a lack of sleep can lead to heart disease. Ongoing sleep deficiency can raise blood pressure, interfere with blood sugar levels, increase levels of stress hormones, and possibly change heart rhythms. So, if you are experiencing sleepless nights, it's important to find ways of getting a good night's sleep, not only because you will feel less fatigued, but because lack of sleep is connected with heart disease.

The following put you at an increased risk for heart disease: high-salt diet, high-fat diet, inactive lifestyle, overweight/obesity or waist measurement >35 inches, smoking, drinking more than one to three alcoholic drinks per day, a family member who died from heart disease prior to the age of 50, diabetes, and difficulty with the body using insulin (insulin resistance).

Many women with heart disease have different symptoms than men. Most of us know that chest pain, especially if it goes down your arm, can be a warning sign of a heart attack. But recently researchers have learned that women can have less commonly recognized symptoms such as fatigue, nausea, poor appetite, neck or back pain, shortness of breath at night, and chest pressure. Since many of these symptoms are experienced in the transition to menopause, it is important to discuss them with your clinician. Appendix A lists resources for detecting and preventing heart disease in women.

45. I've heard that heart disease is not just about the heart. What else does it include, and how is it related to menopause?

Heart disease does not just involve heart attacks. Heart disease includes many conditions related to the heart and blood vessels. See Table 9 for a description of the various forms of heart disease. If you have not yet reached menopause, you are less likely to have heart disease because it is rare in women before menopause (except for high blood pressure). There are several specific changes that may explain some of the increased risk of heart disease after menopause. Insulin levels, blood sugar, and cholesterol levels including total cholesterol, LDL, and triglycerides (sugary fats) increase following menopause, possibly due to lower estrogen levels. Although a daily dose of 81 mg of aspirin has been effective in helping to prevent repeat heart attacks, it's too early to say that every postmenopausal woman should take aspirin regularly to help prevent heart disease.

Estrogen and progesterone have receptors in blood vessels. So, when the hormone levels fall during menopause, the vessels become less elastic and more

Table 9   Types of Heart Disease

Medical Term	Commonly Used Term/Explanation
Angina	pain and pressure in the chest usually associated with narrowing and lack of elasticity of the heart vessels
Arrhythmias or Dysrhythmias	abnormal heart rhythms or irregular heartbeats
Atherosclerosis	hardening of the arteries (an accumulation of plaque deposits of fats and cholesterol that line blood vessels and cause the vessels to narrow and restrict blood flow)
Cardiomyopathy	enlarged heart, can be present from birth or develop later in life due to medications, drugs, or other illnesses (reduces the heart muscle's ability to effectively pump blood through the system)
Congenital heart disease	heart problems that are present at birth (often related to heart enlargement, a faulty heart valve, arrhythmia, or open area between two heart chambers)
Congestive heart failure (CHF)	condition in which the heart can't pump blood effectively to other parts of the body, causes blood to backup in the system
Coronary heart disease (CHD)	narrowing of the arteries of the heart caused by plaque, which is the main reason for myocardial infarctions (heart attacks) and angina
CVA (cardiovascular accident) or stroke	a clot that blocks blood flow in the brain or bleeding of a blood vessel into the brain
Hypertension	high blood pressure
Myocardial infarction	heart attack (area of heart muscle is damaged, caused by reduced or no blood flow to an area of the heart muscle, usually from blood clots or atherosclerosis)
Valvular disease	conditions caused by faulty heart valves (including rheumatic heart disease) that restrict effective blood flow through the heart

constricted. It was once thought that heart disease risk would be reduced by taking hormone therapy after menopause. However, recent research studies have called that into question (see Question 81 about hormone therapy controversy). Hormone therapy is no longer prescribed to prevent heart disease.

46. How do I get tested for heart disease?

You should have your blood pressure checked at least once a year.

You should have your blood pressure checked at least once a year. A normal blood pressure is less than 120/80 mmHg (Hg is the chemical sign for mercury, which was used in the past for measuring blood pressure and temperature). If the top number (the pressure in your system when the heart is beating) is between 120–139 mmHg, and the bottom number (the pressure in the blood vessels when your heart is at rest) is between 80–89 mmHg, you have pre-high blood pressure (prehypertension). If your blood pressure is above 140/90 mmHg, you have high blood pressure (hypertension). Both pre-high blood pressure and high blood pressure need to be treated, usually beginning with lifestyle changes such as reducing salt and exercising, and sometimes medication, as well. Keeping your blood pressure in the normal range is especially important if you have other heart disease risks or diabetes.

Cholesterol testing should be done by the time you are the age of 45, whether you have menopause symptoms or not. The best way to have your cholesterol tested is to do a blood test after you have had nothing to eat or drink except water for at least 8 hours (fasting). If the results show normal cholesterol levels and a low risk for heart disease, you can be tested again in about 5 years. If the levels are high, or you have other risks or get new symptoms, then you may need to have another cholesterol test sooner. The blood test (called a fasting lipid panel) should include all of the cholesterol components:

- Total cholesterol (goal <200 mg/dL)
- HDL [high density lipids or "good" cholesterol] (goal >40 mg/dL)
- LDL [low density lipids or "bad" cholesterol] (goal <130 mg/dL, but <100 mg/dL if at moderate or high risk, or have diabetes or other heart disease)
- Total triglycerides (goal <150 mg/dL)

You can go to the National Heart Lung and Blood Institute web site to calculate your risk for having a heart attack: *http://nhlbi.nih.gov/*.

Some clinicians also recommend having an ECG (electrocardiogram; sometimes called an EKG), which provides a tracing of the electrical activity through the heart muscle. Depending on your symptoms and risk factors, your clinician might also recommend a stress test (treadmill ECG). It's really important to be checked for heart disease before you start a new exercise program, especially if you have diabetes or any of the risks listed in Question 44.

There are things you can do to prevent heart disease from progressing, and to prevent heart attacks. Whether you have higher than normal blood pressure or elevated cholesterol levels, your heart disease may be managed early on with lifestyle changes, such as a heart-healthy diet and more exercise. You need to discuss your lifestyle openly with your clinician. Sometimes, especially when there are other stresses in your personal life, it isn't possible to make big changes in your eating and activity patterns. Your clinician needs to know this so you can work together to manage your health. Even if you can make changes in your eating habits and more, you may need medication. There are several different types of medications available for controlling blood pressure and cholesterol, and each one has possible side effects and risks. It is important to discuss the options with your clinician and read the information from the pharmacist so that you are informed about your medications.

47. What is thyroid disease, and is it more common during menopause?

The thyroid is a gland located at the front of the neck. The thyroid makes thyroid hormones used in the body for growth and metabolism. Although both men and women are more likely to develop thyroid disease as they age, it is more common in women than in men. Screening for thyroid disorders is controversial, but most clinicians suggest a blood test for TSH (thyroid-stimulating hormone) around the age of 40. TSH is not usually tested again unless you have symptoms of high or low levels of thyroid hormones. TSH is tested because it is the hormone that is produced to regulate production of the two main thyroid hormones (T3 and T4). If TSH levels are abnormal, additional tests are done.

Although both men and women are more likely to develop thyroid disease as they age, it is more common in women than in men.

The most common forms of thyroid disease are underactive and overactive thyroid. Underactive thyroid is more common in menopause, but overactive can happen as well. Overactive thyroid (hyperthyroidism) occurs when the thyroid gland produces too much of the thyroid hormones, and is treated with medications and sometimes surgery or radiation. Underactive thyroid (hypothyroidism) occurs when the thyroid gland doesn't produce enough of the thyroid hormones, and is treated with a synthetic thyroid hormone medication. See Table 10, which lists symptoms experienced

Table 10   Signs and Symptoms of Hyperthyroidism and Hypothyroidism

Hyperthyroidism (overactive thyroid gland)	Hypothyroidism (underactive thyroid gland)
Abnormal menstruation—light or absent; infertility	Heavy menstrual periods; infertility
Breathlessness, feeling out of breath during exercise	Weakness
Eye changes (bulging eyes, staring gaze, light sensitivity)	Pale or sallow skin
Fast heart rate/palpitations	Slow heart rate/low body temperature
Fatigue	Fatigue
Frequent bowel movements or diarrhea	Constipation
Hair loss	Coarseness or loss of hair
Inability to tolerate heat	Inability to tolerate cold
Muscle weakness/sudden inability to move	Lack of coordination or balance, poor reflexes
Nervousness	Depression/irritability/memory impairment
Sleep disturbances/insomnia	Decreased sex drive
Thyroid gland enlargement/lump	Thyroid gland enlargement/lump
Tremor, trembling hands	Muscle cramps/aches
Warm, moist skin	Dry, rough, or cold skin
Weight loss/increased appetite	Weight gain or difficulty losing weight

with the two conditions. You can see that many of the symptoms that accompany either over- or underactive thyroid are also symptoms often experienced during perimenopause and menopause, which is why it's so important that you do not assume that your symptoms are "nothing but menopause."

Some women describe the nervousness of overactive thyroid as similar to how they feel if they drink too much caffeine—a jittery feeling with a slight tremor and some sleeplessness. If their heart rate is high, they may also feel out of breath even with everyday activities. It is extremely important to have your thyroid checked if you go to your clinician for depression. Underactive thyroid can mimic the symptoms of depression. Many women like to blame their weight gain on an underactive thyroid, but in fact hypothyroidism is rarely the reason for weight gain. See Question 22 about weight gain.

It is extremely important to have your thyroid checked if you go to your clinician for depression.

48. What is a fibroid, and is it related to menopause?

Fibroids are also called leiomyomas, and are non-cancerous tumors of the uterus. More than half a million women have their uterus removed every year. The American College of Obstetricians and Gynecologists says that 40% of these surgeries are due to fibroids. Fibroids are more common as women age until menopause; after menopause, fibroids are less common.

Fibroids can grow without any symptoms, but they can also cause bothersome symptoms such as lower abdominal and pelvic pain and pressure, pain with intercourse, and abnormal bleeding. Pain and pressure depend on where the fibroid is located. For example, if a woman's fibroid is low down on the uterus wall, it is likely that she will have pain and pressure on her bladder. Fibroids can also cause urine incontinence because they push on the wall of the bladder.

Fibroids will develop in one in three African-American women, and one in five white women. They tend to grow slowly, going from very small to the size of a grapefruit or cantaloupe. They are less common in smokers because of lower levels of estrogen found in women who smoke. They are more common in women who are overweight or obese, and in women who started their periods early and have never been pregnant.

Although most fibroids shrink in response to the low estrogen levels found after menopause, some do not. If the fibroid continues to increase in size, it may be found during a regular pelvic examination when the clinician feels the uterus. If the uterus is larger than usual, the clinician will do a pregnancy test first to be certain you aren't pregnant. The next step is usually an ultrasound of the uterus, called a transvaginal ultrasound because the ultrasound wand is placed in the vagina during the test so the uterus and ovaries can be seen better. Sometimes a CT scan is needed to see the fibroid better.

The symptoms a woman experiences depend on both the size and location of the fibroid. The symptoms can be subtle at first but may grow in severity as the fibroid itself grows. Symptoms might include intestinal pressure, constipation, backache, pain with intercourse, infertility, miscarriage, premature labor, enlarged abdomen, and urinary frequency, urgency, retention, or incontinence. If large enough, fibroids can affect other organs as well, such as blocking normal urine flow from the kidneys.

Fibroids can also cause abnormal bleeding, like excessively heavy periods, prolonged and heavy periods, or bleeding between periods. Your clinician must evaluate abnormal bleeding. Sometimes the bleeding will be the first symptom of a fibroid. But even if you know you have a fibroid, abnormal bleeding needs to be checked out. Don't just assume it is your fibroid. In some instances, abnormal bleeding can be heavy enough to cause anemia.

Even if you know you have a fibroid, abnormal bleeding needs to be checked out.

Treatment for fibroids focuses on minimizing the symptoms and controlling bleeding. Usually medications are tried first, but a hysterectomy may still be necessary. In most cases, hormones in very low doses can correct the bleeding without increasing the size of the fibroid, and may even help decrease the size. Another option for treatment can be a progestin-containing IUD. If you are treated with GnRH (gonadotropin-releasing hormone) to curb estrogen production and shrink the size of your fibroid, the side effects can include many of the usual symptoms of perimenopause and menopause.

If you don't have symptoms, surgery is usually not necessary. But if you do need surgery, the fibroid alone might be removed (called a myomectomy), or the entire uterus will be removed (hysterectomy). If you have completed childbearing, hysterectomy is the most common surgery for fibroids. Endometrial ablation (removal of the endometrial tissue) is done only rarely to control bleeding. A newer option is also available, called fibroid embolization, where tiny bits of a plastic material are put into the blood vessel that leads to the fibroid. The tiny bits of plastic eventually cut off the blood supply to the fibroid so that it shrinks and dies off.

The size of a newly identified fibroid is usually evaluated every few months with exams by a clinician and with ultrasounds. If the size stays the same or has a very slow increase, the time between checks can be extended to 6 months. A rapid increase in the size of the fibroid can be a sign of an extremely rare form of cancer.

Pamela's comment:

On top of everything else I am dealing with a fibroid—they tell me not to worry, it is an "innocent" tumor. Who ever heard of any tumor being innocent? He said I can just have my uterus removed if the bleeding gets too bad—but I don't really want surgery. I am kind of partial to keeping my body parts, thank you. So instead, I have amazing cramps, heavy, heavy bleeding, and I really feel drained. On top of that I am moody and not getting any sleep. What's next?!

49. Can I still get pregnant before my periods have stopped for a full year?

Yes, absolutely, you can get pregnant during that time and at any other time during perimenopause. While you might not have a period for several months, your periods can begin again unexpectedly. You can only depend on being in menopause once you have not menstruated for a full 12 months, which you really only know in hindsight. Since ovulation happens about

14 days before menstruation, there's always a chance that you're ovulating even if you haven't had your period for 11 months.

Some women will never have irregular periods and will just stop having periods for that full year. But it is impossible to predict exactly when you will have your final menstrual period. And until you do, it is still possible to become pregnant.

Women who are in perimenopause, which includes the menopause transition as well as the year you have not had periods, have the second highest rate of unintended pregnancy (adolescent girls have the highest rate at 95%). Seventy-seven percent of women between the ages of 40 and 44 who get pregnant do not intend to become pregnant. If you do become pregnant during perimenopause, it doesn't mean that you've done something wrong. Condoms can break, diaphragms can become dislodged, you could forget to take a pill, or your body can simply have a different response to your birth control method.

Even though your method of birth control or natural family planning (ovulation awareness, rhythm method, etc.) has worked for many years, your body can respond differently to the method, and that method may prove unreliable during perimenopause. For example, if you have been on birth control pills for 10 years without pregnancy or bothersome side effects, you may suddenly develop breakthrough bleeding. The pill has not changed, but your body's response to it has. This does not mean that you should stop taking it, but it does mean that you should see your clinician to see if you need a change of prescription. Natural family planning is especially difficult during perimenopause due to the variations and unpredictability in cycles. Other, more effective methods are recommended instead.

If you skip a period, the first thing you should do is get a pregnancy test. More than likely, you have the irregular periods of perimenopause. But the sooner you know if you're pregnant, the better.

If you skip a period, the first thing you should do is get a pregnancy test.

50. What types of birth control should I use?

There are many types of contraception that you can use while you're going through perimenopause. See Table 11 for a listing of birth control methods with their advantages and disadvantages. A frank discussion with your clinician about the best method for you should include the following issues:

- *Fertility*: Are you still interested in having children at a later time?
- *Permanence*: Are you finished having children and ready to prevent pregnancy permanently?
- *Body comfort*: Are you comfortable with inserting a diaphragm or vaginal ring?
- *Frequency and spontaneity of intercourse*: Do you want a method that is reliable but doesn't require diaphragm insertion or condom placement prior to intimacy? Is it worth it to you to take daily birth control pills even if you might have infrequent intercourse?
- *Confidence in being on hormones*: Birth control pills contain higher doses of estrogen and progesterone than the estrogen-progestin therapy given to manage menopausal symptoms. Several studies have

Table 11 Birth Control Methods

Type of Birth Control	Advantages	Disadvantages
Birth Control Pills (Oral Contraception) Estrogen-progestin Combinations* (Alesse, Loestrin, Ovcon-35, Nordette, Lo Ovral, Demulen, Yasmin, Ortho-Cept, EstrostepFe, Triphasil, others)	Highly effective against pregnancy; get benefits of being on hormones—can decrease perimenopausal symptoms such as moodiness, irregular or heavy periods, and hot flashes; supports bone density; easy administration.	Contraindicated in women >35 who smoke due to clotting; may be contraindicated in those with hypertension or diabetes; contraindicated in those with history of migraines, breast cancer, or blood clots; some antibiotics can interfere with effectiveness; must remember one pill per day; can't tell when menopause happens.
IUDs (Intrauterine Devices) Progestin-Containing (Mirena) or plain (copper T)	Good for those with heavy bleeding and with fibroids; progestin-containing IUDs can be used with estrogen therapy for endometrial protection against overgrowth or cancer; very effective method of birth control.	Not as easy to insert in women who have not had children; doesn't give regularity of cycles associated with estrogen-progestin combinations because body hormone production continues.
Diaphragms	No hormones; used with spermicide which, if it contains nonoxyl-9, is most effective against HIV infection.	Correct size must be fitted by clinician; less effective without spermicide (women sometimes develop reactions to spermicide during perimenopause); reduces spontaneity because must be inserted prior to intercourse.

Table 11 Birth Control Methods (continued)

Type of Birth Control	Advantages	Disadvantages
Condoms	Both male and female types available, female condom affords more protection because the "wings" of the condom cover the labia (vaginal "lips"); available with ribbing or flavors that may enhance sexual pleasure; no hormones; protects against many sexually transmitted infections; used with spermicide which, if it contains nonoxyl-9, is most effective against HIV infection.	Allergies or skin irritation from latex and spermicide; reduces spontaneity because must be applied prior to intercourse.
Vaginal Ring– (NuvaRing)	Worn in vagina; self-inserted; worn for 3 weeks, none for 1 week then new ring placed; very effective method of birth control; get benefits of being on hormones.	If it falls out, only a 3-hour "window of protection;" must be comfortable enough with body to put it in yourself.
Rod Implant (Implanon) soon to be released	Implanted in skin of upper arm; replaced every 2 to 3 years; provides immediate contraception; return to fertility occurs in 1 to 3 months after removal; similar effectiveness and side-effects as oral contraceptive pills; contains low-dose progestin only.	Irregular bleeding can occur; minor office procedure needed for insertion and removal.
Depo-Provera Injection** (progestin)	Works for several months; doesn't require remembering (except for appointments for injection every 3 months).	Not a good choice if you want to become pregnant within one year or if you are queasy about shots; long-term use may increase risk of bone loss.

Table 11 Birth Control Methods (continued)

Type of Birth Control	Advantages	Disadvantages
Patch (Ortho-Evra)	One patch on for 3 weeks, no patch for one week then new patch; as effective as oral pills with same advantages; only have to remember patch every 7 days; decreases the nausea sometimes associated with oral contraceptives.	Not to be used in women who weigh over 198 pounds (due to lower effectiveness); same contraindications as oral pills; watch for sensitivity to adhesive.
Natural Family Planning	Preferred by some religious doctrines; no hormones are absorbed or ingested.	Ovulation more difficult to predict with changes of mucus, libido, and mood; rhythm method is unreliable when periods become irregular; basal body temperature also unreliable due to fluctuations in hormones and the ease with which body temperature changes; not recommended for perimenopausal women.
Sterilization Male: vasectomy Female: Tubal ligation or Transcervical sterilizataion (Essure)	*Vasectomy:* reliable *Tubal ligation:* nonhormonal method, woman knows when she has reached menopause. *Essure* method uses a tiny coil inserted through the cervix into each fallopian tube, which scars over and blocks the tube. It can be done under local anesthesia in an office setting. Permanent methods of birth control should only be considered by those who are done having children.	All surgical procedures carry risks. Tubal ligation is not as reliable as oral contraception, IUDs, or vasectomy at preventing pregnancy. Essure method is not effective immediately. All methods of surgical sterilization are considered nonreversible.

Table 11 Birth Control Methods (continued)

Type of Birth Control	Advantages	Disadvantages
Sponge (dome shaped soft sponge with spermicide imbedded in it)	No hormones; has spermicide in it already; soon to be available in drug stores in the United States; one size fits all, no fitting needed.	Women sometimes develop reactions to spermicide during perimenopause; reduces spontaneity because must be inserted prior to intercourse.

*Progestin-only pills are also available, they often cause irregular bleeding at first but later most women have no periods, they may be a good option for women who are sensitive to estrogens. Examples of progestin-only pills are Micronor, Nor-QD, Ovrette.

demonstrated a protective effect against ovarian and endometrial cancer. If you opt for taking the pill, you will not only have a highly effective method for contraception, you will likely go through perimenopause and into postmenopause with fewer hot flashes. See Question 52 about being on birth control pills and wondering if you're in menopause.

- *Number of partners*: Do you need added protection from **sexually transmitted infections** such as gonorrhea, **chlamydia**, syphilis, trichomoniasis, and HIV?
- *Your confidence in remembering things*: Will you be able to remember to take a pill every day or change a patch every week?

In addition to the advantages and disadvantages listed in Table 11, there are some other considerations for birth control during perimenopause including the transition year after your final menstrual period:

- While family planning and fertility awareness methods may have worked in the past, the fluctuation and unpredictability of hormone levels makes it difficult to rely on these methods to avoid pregnancy.
- Withdrawal (coitus interruptus), where the male partner withdraws prior to ejaculation, is not a reliable method of birth control because pre-ejaculatory fluid can contain sperm, especially when it is the second ejaculate in a row.
- Breastfeeding, believed historically to be effective in preventing pregnancy, is not a reliable method of birth control. There is some controversy over how long breastfeeding curbs estrogen production. If you are breastfeeding exclusively (no supplements or solid food for the baby), you can rely on this

Sexually transmitted infections

formerly called sexually transmitted diseases. Infections contracted during sexual contact. Such infections include herpes, gonorrhea, syphilis, human immunodeficiency virus (HIV), several forms of hepatitis including B and C, and chlamydia.

Chlamydia

a common bacterial infection transmitted vaginally, orally, or anally during sex that can often have no symptoms. It can cause burning and inflammation of the urethra, and vaginal discharge. It can lead to infertility if untreated.

method of birth control for about 3 months after the baby is born. Some clinicians advise their patients to always use a barrier method of birth control (diaphragm, condom) in case they ovulate while breastfeeding.

- Should you choose a permanent method of birth control, a bilateral tubal ligation, which is a surgical interruption of the fallopian tubes, is generally considered irreversible. There is about a 5% failure rate with this method, and there is also the risk of tubal pregnancy. The new permanent sterilization method called Essure carries fewer surgical risks for the woman, but is not effective for at least 3 months after the small coil is inserted into each fallopian tube. A **vasectomy** for your male partner is associated with fewer surgical risks than traditional tubal ligation and is highly effective.

- Although emergency contraception should not be considered an ongoing method of birth control, there are two formulations that can be taken by mouth in the event of unprotected intercourse or an unanticipated exposure such as a broken condom or dislodged diaphragm. Preven® (estrogen and progestin) or Plan B® (progestin only) can be taken up to 5 days after unprotected intercourse. Nausea and vomiting side effects are more likely with the products that contain estrogen. Emergency contraception is currently only available by prescription, but it may become available without a prescription in the future.

Vasectomy
the surgery that cuts the vas deferens, the connection from the testis to the urethra in a male, so that sperm cannot be part of the ejaculate.

51. How is menopause diagnosed? Is FSH testing needed?

Menopause can only be definitively diagnosed once you have experienced 12 months without any menstrual periods. Once those 12 months are up, you can be almost 100% certain that you have reached menopause. It is extremely rare for a woman to begin to have periods again once those 12 months are over, except in special circumstances where menopause was induced temporarily by a medical condition or chemotherapy (see Question 13 about induced menopause).

Testing FSH (follicle-stimulating hormone) levels in the blood is no longer considered an accurate method of diagnosing menopause. You will recall that FSH responds to low levels of estrogen, and it was believed that once FSH stayed very high, this meant that the ovary was no longer putting out estrogen, and you were therefore headed for menopause. Now that we know that FSH levels are unpredictable based on whether the ovary secretes estrogen, testing for it no longer makes sense. Some clinicians test FSH repeatedly, and if it is consistently high (above 40 international units per milliliter) see it as an indication that a woman is in menopause. But even if a woman does not get her period for 6 months and her FSH levels are consistently high, there is still no way to predict for sure if the ovary will suddenly secrete estrogen, giving her a period in the seventh month. Other hormone levels are also not routinely tested for the diagnosis of menopause. See Figure 13, which shows the erratic levels of FSH and estrogen during perimenopause.

Over-the-counter kits that measure FSH levels in the urine have recently appeared on drugstore shelves. The premise of these home kits is that you can diagnose menopause in the privacy of your own bathroom. However, no urine test can accurately diagnose that you are in menopause unless you have not had your

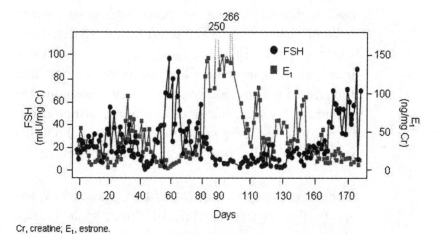

Cr, creatine; E₁, estrone.

Figure 13   Follicle-stimulating hormone (FSH) and estrogen levels during perimenopause. (Reprinted with permission from Warner Chilcott, Inc.)

period for 12 months. By the time you have missed your period for 12 months in a row, you already know you are in menopause, so the kits won't tell you anything new. The home kits for menopause should not be used as pregnancy tests, either.

52. I'm taking birth control pills. How do I know if I've reached menopause?

Many women use birth control pills, patches, or rings after menopause as long as they don't smoke and do not have health problems. If you are taking birth control pills the traditional way (21 active pills followed by 7 hormone-free pills), you will be having regular cycles. This means that you will not miss your periods for the necessary 12 months to identify menopause. Birth control pills contain more than enough estrogen to prevent you from experiencing hot flashes, night sweats, vaginal dryness, or other bothersome symptoms of menopause, so you won't be able to determine whether you're in menopause based on the usual menopausal symptoms. The converse is not true though: HT does not contain enough hormones to prevent pregnancy, but does relieve the symptoms of menopause. So, how will you know if your body has stopped making its own estrogen and progesterone?

There are a couple of ways of figuring out where you are in the menopause timeline. First, some women choose to go off birth control pills for a few months to see if they are still menstruating on their own. They will need to use a nonhormonal method of birth control until menopause is determined. In order to avoid being off birth control pills for a full year, or to go on and off birth control pills to see if menstruation returns on its own, clinicians may, in this case, choose to do repeated FSH levels to see if they are consistently elevated. Women must be off hormones for at least 2 weeks before the FSH can be accurately measured. If the levels remain above 40 for three consecutive measures, it's safe to say that the woman has reached menopause if she is around 51 years of age (the average age of menopause). However, most women won't relish the idea of going off birth control pills just to see what will happen. So, it is more common for clinicians to keep a woman on the lowest possible dose of birth control pills with the fewest side effects until she can transition over to HT. Some clinicians recommend making the transition at the age of 51, the average age of menopause. Other clinicians will wait until the woman is between 53 and 55.

53. When should I get my symptoms evaluated? How will I know if my symptoms are related to other medical conditions and not menopause?

There are recommendations for yearly health screenings for women age 40 and over, such as mammograms and blood pressure checks. See Table 3 (page 67), which lists screening tests that are recommended for midlife women. When you have a routine visit with your primary care clinician or your gynecology clinician, you should always discuss the symptoms that you are experiencing, whether they feel severe or not, because menopause symptoms can mimic several other midlife health problems.

There are some perimenopausal symptoms that should not wait for a routine checkup, including abnormal or irregular menstrual bleeding; palpitations or shortness of breath; excessive fatigue; difficulty with concentration; or any symptom that interferes with your ability to participate in and enjoy daily life.

You may be able to manage some symptoms that you find bothersome, but they might also require a visit to your clinician. Your clinician may have additional suggestions, or may refer you to a specialist or someone more knowledgeable about menopause. You should never just stay at home feeling tired and "crummy," and thinking that there's nothing that can be done for you. Most symptoms can be managed and you *can* feel better. See Parts 4 and 5 about treatment options for your menopausal symptoms.

Most symptoms can be managed and you can feel better.

Sometimes women have perimenopausal symptoms that are worse because medical problems are not controlled. For example, you might be experiencing hot flashes, difficulty sleeping, and fatigue that you believe is related to menopause. Yet, at your yearly physical you find out that you have diabetes and high blood pressure. Once your blood pressure and blood sugar are controlled, your hot flashes and fatigue might go away—or at least be less severe.

Cherise's comment:

I was having terrible flashes, I felt hot and got all sweated out. It was disgusting. I went to get checked at my gyno for the hot flashes because this one sister at church thought it was menopause, but the blood pressure was very high, almost at stroke level, and I was not even aware of it. Yeah, the blood pressure was up… that's what it was. Once he put me on the blood pressure medicine the hot flashes stopped. That was it.

PART FOUR

Lifestyle Changes and Alternative Therapies

What are phytoestrogens? Are they the same as natural hormones?

Are there other herbs that would be helpful in treating my symptoms?

Is there a special "menopause diet"? What foods will help me stay healthy at midlife?

What would help me sleep better?

Will regular exercise help my symptoms? What kind of exercise is most appropriate during menopause?

More ...

54. I've heard that some complementary and alternative therapies are helpful in the treatment of menopausal symptoms. Is that true?

Yes, some women find complementary and alternative therapies very helpful for menopausal symptoms. **Complementary therapies** are therapies or practices used with conventional medical treatments. **Alternative therapies** are therapies or practices used in place of conventional medical treatments. Many people use both alternative and conventional medical therapies at the same time. There are several categories of complementary and alternative therapies identified by the National Center for Complementary and Alternative Medicine (a division of the National Institutes of Health):

- *Alternative medical systems* such as homeopathic medicine, naturopathic medicine, and **acupuncture**.
- *Mind-body interventions* such as **guided imagery**, prayer, cognitive therapy, hypnosis, and support groups.
- *Biologically based therapies* such as herbal treatments (e.g., black cohosh) and **dietary supplements** (e.g., **phytoestrogens,** progesterone creams).
- *Manipulative and body-based methods* such as chiropractic, massage, acupressure, and aromatherapy.
- *Energy therapies* such as Therapeutic Touch and the use of magnets.

Despite conflicting research reports, many women report relief from hot flashes, stress, and poor sleep

Complementary therapies

therapies or practices used with conventional medical treatments.

Acupuncture

a form of alternative medicine that uses tiny needles inserted along qi (energy) lines (meridians).

Mind-body interventions

any therapy or process engaged in to use the mind as a healing tool for the body.

Guided imagery

a process used to help someone imagine a picture or a place. It is used during psychotherapy as a way to focus on problems or during uncomfortable procedures like chemotherapy to divert attention away from pain and nausea. It is also commonly used to assist with relaxation (e.g., imagining a gentle stream with ducks floating on it).

from a variety of complementary and alternative therapies. And, the use of complementary and alternative therapies is on the rise among women in the United States. It is very important that you tell your clinician if you are using any of these therapies, some of which can compound or interfere with prescription hormones and medications. It is also important to learn what might be of use for your own circumstances, so that you can make an informed decision about these types of therapies.

Jackie's comment:

A friend was going through menopause at the same time as I was and we decided to go the herbal route. The book we bought about herbs basically helped us develop a more positive attitude—that the changes of menopause don't have to be negative. We learned that we could get through it best if we had a good outlook. I had some rough spots but I was done by the time I was 41 or 42 with my hot flashes and I'm 50 now. I learned how to deal best with my hot flashes—if I was hot, I opened the window! I would advise taking your multivitamin, take your calcium, and be careful of caffeine.

55. What are phytoestrogens? Are they the same as natural hormones?

Phytoestrogens are weak, estrogen-like substances found in plants, but they are not the same as "natural" hormones, which can also be made from plants. (See Question 85 for more information about bio-identical hormones.) Natural hormones are made from a steroid molecule found in **wild yam** and soy. Phytoestrogens are complex compounds that are converted into weak, estrogen-like substances by the bacteria that live in your intestines.

Alternative therapies
therapies or practices used in place of conventional medical treatments.

Dietary supplement
any substance that is added to the diet, such as vitamins, minerals, or herbs, in addition to what your body already takes in. Some progesterone creams are also termed dietary supplements even though you don't eat them.

Phytoestrogens
weak, estrogen-like substances that are in plants. Can be eaten in whole foods, such as soy, or extracted from red clover in the form of isoflavones and made into supplements.

Wild yam
an herb that was originally used to manufacture progesterone starting in the 1940s. It does not contain progesterone, but instead contains a molecule that is used to manufacture progesterone in a laboratory.

Isoflavones are the phytoestrogens that are most commonly used for menopausal symptoms.

There are several major groups of phytoestrogens that are commonly found in foods. Isoflavones are the phytoestrogens that are most commonly used for menopausal symptoms. They are found in legumes such as soybeans, and also occur naturally in red clover and kudzu. Your body can absorb isoflavones when you eat foods that contain them or when you take dietary supplements that contain them. Isoflavones in dietary supplements are extracted from plants and manufactured into tablets or capsules, like Promensil™ or Rimostil™.

The isoflavones found in soy protein and those found in clover are different from each other. They are also different from those found in whole grains and fruits like red grapes. After you eat tofu (soybean curd) or a whole grain cereal, or drink a glass of red wine, your intestines digest and change these plant chemicals into substances that can act like estrogen in your body.

Several recent studies of phytoestrogens, extracted from soy and/or red clover and manufactured in tablet form, showed disappointing results for controlling menopausal hot flashes. But other studies have shown some benefits. Conflicting research reports aside, many women who take isoflavone preparations such as Promensil™ and Rimostil™ do report a reduction in hot flashes. Soy is a heart-healthy food, and isoflavones may also have some positive effects on bones and "good" cholesterol (HDL). So, go ahead and try soy or isoflavones for your symptoms.

56. Is it safe for me to take phytoestrogens?

Phytoestrogens are weak, estrogen-like substances that are generally believed to be safe when taken in moderate amounts, either alone or as a supplement to other estrogen therapies.

Phytoestrogens in the form of tablets and capsules can be bought without prescription and are considered dietary supplements. Dosages can vary depending on the manufacturer, and your body may absorb each type of isoflavone differently. It takes about 100 grams of soy protein to make 97 mg of isoflavones, but the amount of soy protein in various foods differs, and how your body uses the isoflavones may be different as well. The FDA agrees that 25 grams of soy protein per day can be beneficial to heart health by reducing cholesterol levels. But they did not have enough evidence to comment on a specific amount of isoflavone that should be in the 25 grams of soy.

Eating phytoestrogen-containing soy products, whole grains, fruits, vegetables, and flax seed is not only healthy, but may provide you with some relief from menopausal symptoms. Japanese women tend to have a high soy diet, fewer menopausal symptoms, and lower rates of breast cancer, all of which suggests that phytoestrogens may have several health benefits.

Whether isoflavones help protect bones is another important consideration. Although Japanese women are at higher risk for bone loss than American women, some small studies suggest that isoflavones may protect bone strength. We don't know enough yet to say for sure. We also don't know enough about their effect on the uterine lining. Some studies show that they do not cause overgrowth, but other studies indicate they can contribute to overgrowth if taken for 5 years or longer. The long-term safety and effects of isoflavones on bones, breasts, heart, and menopause symptoms are currently being studied, so keep an eye out for more information that you can use to make an informed choice for treatment.

The conflicting research doesn't mean that soy, phytoestrogens, and herbs are unsafe, or that they can't relieve hot flashes in individual women. Furthermore, since soy has been identified as a heart-healthy food, it is a great food to include in your diet.

57. You mentioned black cohosh among the alternative therapies. Would you recommend taking it for hot flashes? I've heard that I cannot take black cohosh for longer than 6 months. Is that true, and are there any side effects I should look for?

Black cohosh (*Actaea racemosa* or *Cimicifuga racemosa*), also called black snakeroot, bugwort, bugbane, rattleroot, rattletop, macrotys, and squawroot, is an herb in the buttercup family used frequently in Native American medicine for a variety of ailments including rheumatism, colds, constipation, backache, and gynecological disorders. A preparation of black cohosh (Remifemin Menopause®) has been available in Europe for over 40 years and is now widely available in the United States.

The American College of Obstetricians and Gynecologists agreed in 2001 that black cohosh may be helpful in the treatment of hot flashes. And some small studies have shown that it reduces hot flashes in women. Even so, many clinicians are skeptical because there have not been large long-term research studies yet that prove it. Two big clinical trials sponsored by the National Center for Complementary and Alternative Medicine are under way to look at the use of black cohosh for up to 1 year. Researchers in these studies are checking hot flashes, hormone levels, and effects on the uterine lining.

Black cohosh can be purchased at drug stores and health food stores. Capsules contain from 60 to 545 mg, and tablets contain between 60 and 120 mg. It is often combined with other herbs, phytoestrogens, and vitamins or minerals to make a tablet that is advertised for the relief of menopausal symptoms or for hormonal balance. For example, Estroven® contains black cohosh, date seed, magnolia bark, several B vitamins, selenium, calcium, and isoflavones from soy, just to name a few ingredients.

Black cohosh is not advised when you're taking estrogen or estrogen-progestin therapies. Black cohosh is not a phytoestrogen, but it might have some estrogen-like activity in the body and does have the same contraindications for use as estrogen (see Question 78 about when to avoid estrogen therapy). As with hormone therapy or any therapy, you should use the smallest dose possible to get relief from your symptoms.

The safety record for taking black cohosh up to 6 months is good. But doses vary among different preparations, and the higher doses have not been studied. Some preparations are made with only 20 mg, others with 333 mg, and still others with 545 mg. Women taking the higher doses have reported some side effects like headache and stomach upset. Heaviness in the legs and low blood pressure are other possible side effects. There have also been a few cases of hepatitis (inflammation of the liver) reported in women taking black cohosh.

You should not take black cohosh if you already take medication for high blood pressure, because it can have an added effect and lower your blood pressure too much. Black cohosh is not the same as blue cohosh, which has been used to increase menstrual flow, and may have heart and intestinal side effects.

We don't yet know the long-term effects from taking black cohosh, but short-term use may be worth a try. Exactly how black cohosh works is not completely understood, so it is not clear whether it has estrogen-like activity, or whether it can affect breast tissue.

Gayle's comment:

For 7 years I took HT for menopause. In 2003 my doctor recommended I stop taking it. Immediately my hot flashes and night/day sweats started up again. With so many alternative therapies on the market these days, I decided to research some of them. Black cohosh seemed to be the main ingredient in several over-the-counter therapies I looked at. After reading about it on the web I decided to try it. Normally you can expect to see results in 10–14 days. I took the recommended dosage of 20 mg at night and in the morning. After a week I started feeling normal again and continued to take it for about 7–8 months without any hot flashes or sweating. During that time I continued to research it while touting its merits to everyone who would listen. However, everything I read suggested that it not be taken for more than 6 months. Reluctantly, I decided to discontinue using it and secretly hoped I didn't need it anymore anyway. Wrong! All my old symptoms came back. While I haven't taken anything to curb my symptoms since then, I firmly believe black cohosh got me through a difficult time in my life, even if for only a short time.

58. Are there other herbs that would be helpful in treating my symptoms?

There are many products with red clover (*Trifolium pratense*) that are advertised to help with menopause symptoms, but scientific evidence about whether red clover as an herb helps relieve hot flashes is conflicting. Isoflavones made from red clover are different from red clover itself. See Questions 55 and 56 about phytoestrogens and isoflavones made from red clover and soy.

Chastetree (*Vitex agnus castus*) has been used to treat "menstrual cycle irregularities" for many years in Germany, but has not been studied for its specific effects on menopause. Dong quai (*Angelica sinensis*) is an herb that is often used in combination with other herbs in the practice of Chinese medicine. Dong quai has not been found to be effective in treating menopause symptoms.

Kava (*Piper methysticum*) has been used around the world to reduce anxiety and help with sleep. But some countries have recently banned Kava because of its possible toxic effects on the liver. St. John's wort (*Hypericum perforatum*), long used to treat depression, has not been studied to see if it has positive effects on menopause symptoms. St. John's wort does reach high enough blood levels to interfere with the effects of several prescription medications, including birth control pills.

Ginseng (*panax ginseng*) did not show benefits for hot flashes or vaginal symptoms but did improve depression, well being, and general health in a randomized, controlled trial of 384 patients. Ginseng is often available in a mixture with other herbs and substances, so it is important to read labels carefully. It is not to be used by those who have breast cancer.

Dementia

condition marked by memory loss, lack of ability to attend to personal care, personality changes, impaired reasoning, and bouts of disorientation.

Ginkgo (*ginkgo biloba*) is an herb that many think will slow the progress of **dementia**; one large study supports this belief. But so far, there have been no studies evaluating whether gingko will help menopausal women who are experiencing forgetfulness.

Licorice (*glycyrrhiza glabra*) is used in many combination products made for menopausal symptom relief. There is no evidence that it works on menopausal symptoms, and in very high doses it can be dangerous. (Licorice candy does not contain the licorice herb.)

Always tell your clinician about all herbs or dietary supplements you decide you would like to try.

You may be under the assumption that if you're taking an herb or dietary supplement, you are not taking anything harmful because it's "natural." But just as drugs interact with each other, and even grapefruit juice can interfere with the absorption of certain medications, herbs and dietary supplements can reduce the effect or increase the blood levels of some prescription or nonprescription medications. Always tell your clinician about all herbs or dietary supplements you decide you would like to try. See Table 12 for more information on some herbs used for menopause-related concerns.

Lifestyle Changes and Alternative Therapies

Table 12   Herbals Used Commonly for Menopause Symptom Relief*

Herb	Potential Use	Comments
Black cohosh (*Actaea racemosa* or *Cimicifuga racemosa*)	• Hot flashes	• Menopausal symptoms • Many products and formulations available • Ingredients, purity, manufacturing processes can vary • Helpful for menopausal symptoms • Safety for using longer than 6 months not known • Do not use if taking medicine for high blood pressure • Side effects rare, usually stomach upset, headache, dizziness, low blood pressure or pain in arms or legs; more common with higher doses
Chastetree berry (*Vitex agnus castus*)	• Menstrual irregularity	• More popular in Europe than in the United States • May prompt progesterone production by body • Often in combination products • Helpful for PMS symptoms, no information on menopause • Side effects rare, usually headache, stomach upset, tired, and hair loss • Do not use if you are taking birth control pills or have irregular bleeding
Dong quai (*Angelica sinensis*)	• Gynecologic conditions	• Popular in Asia • Research found no benefit for menopause symptoms • Given in combination Chinese herb products, not alone • Do not use if you take blood thinners • Side effects include sensitivity to light, low blood pressure, red face, hot flashes, sweating, irritability, or difficulty sleeping

131

Table 12 Herbals Used Commonly for Menopause Symptom Relief* (continued)

Herb	Potential Use	Comments
Evening primrose oil (*Oenothera biennis*)	• Hot flashes • Breast pain	• Research found no benefit for hot flashes • Do not use if you have a seizure disorder or are taking blood thinners • Side-effects include diarrhea, nausea, headaches, blood clots; risk increases if use for >1 year • Oil is used in a botanical mixture (Zestra) for increasing sexual function and pleasure in women
Ginkgo (*Ginkgo biloba*)	• Memory changes	• Helps slow advancement of Alzheimer's disease and dementia • Do not use if you take blood thinners • Effect on memory changes in menopause unknown • Side effects include stomach upset, low blood pressure; long-term use linked with bleeding problems
Ginseng (*Panax ginseng*)	• General "tonic" • Mood changes • Fatigue • Difficulty with concentration	• Used in combination products • Many forms of ginseng (American, Brazilian, Chinese, Korean, and Siberian) • Helpful for well-being, general health, and depression; no benefit on menopausal symptoms • Use with care if you have diabetes or heart disease • Do not use if you have breast cancer • Many medicine interactions, review possible medicine interactions with your clinician before taking • Side effects include uterine bleeding, breast pain, rash, nervousness, insomnia, hypertension

Table 12   Herbals Used Commonly for Menopause Symptom Relief* (continued)

Herb	Potential Use	Comments
Kava (*Piper methysticum*)	• Irritability • Insomnia	• Not recommended because can cause liver damage; banned in several countries • Can be addicting • Do not use with alcohol or if you have depression • Side effects include stomach pain, rash, slowed reflexes and movement, weight loss, liver damage
Licorice root (*Glycyrrhiza glabra*)	• Menopause-related symptoms	• Research found no benefit for hot flashes • Used in combination products • Active ingredients are phytoestrogens (isoflavones and lignans) • High doses linked with heart attack, irregular heart rhythms, adrenal gland disorder • Do not use if you have kidney or liver disease, diabetes, high blood pressure, heart rhythm disorders, low potassium levels, high muscle tension, are pregnant, or taking water pills (diuretics)
Passion flower (*Passiflora incarnata*)	• Insomnia	• Research shows mixed results in sleep improvement • Found in combination with valerian as a sleep aid • Sleep disturbance in menopause often due to hot flashes, sweats, or stress • Do not use if you are taking an MAO inhibitor

Table 12   Herbals Used Commonly for Menopause Symptom Relief* (continued)

Herb	Potential Use	Comments
Red clover (*Trifolium pratense*)	• Hot flashes	• Research shows mixed results in hot flash relief • Isoflavones are often isolated from red clover • Do not use if you are taking estrogen, progesterone, or blood thinners, or if you are pregnant or have breast cancer • Long-term effects not known • High doses can cause rash
St John's wort (*Hypericum perforatum*)	• Hot flashes • Irritability • Depression	• Helpful for depression; no information for menopause • Often combined with black cohosh for menopause symptom treatment • Many medicine interactions, review possible medicine interactions with your clinician before taking • Side effects include rash, sun sensitivity, constipation, cramping, dry mouth, tired, dizzy, restless, sleep disturbances
Valerian root (*Valeriana officinalis*)	• Insomnia • Anxiety	• Helpful for sleep disturbances, depression, anxiety • May take 2 weeks or more to be effective for sleep • Do not drive or use machines while taking Valerian • Do not use with other sedatives • Side effects include headache, uneasiness, excitability, irregular heart rhythms, morning tiredness, stomach upset, heart problems (with long-term use)

Table 12   Herbals Used Commonly for Menopause Symptom Relief* (continued)

Herb	Potential Use	Comments
Wild yam (*Dioscorea villosa*)	• Menopausal symptoms	• Research found no benefit for menopausal symptoms • Products claim that creams are converted to progesterone, but the human body cannot convert wild yam into progesterone

*You should not take any herbs unless you have had a recent physical exam to determine if any of your symptoms are part of medical conditions unrelated to perimenopause and menopause. The concentration of herbs varies by how they're taken, e.g., by liquid extracts, drops, essential oils, standardized extract, or tea-type infusions. Not all clinicians will be comfortable giving advice about herbs. You may need to consult a licensed herbalist, naturopathic physician, or holistic practitioner for advice about the use of herbs for treating your menopausal symptoms.

59. What about Vitamin E, and other vitamins and minerals? Should I be taking a daily vitamin supplement?

There are several benefits to dietary Vitamin E. It acts as an **antioxidant** to prevent cell damage, may help to prevent Alzheimer's and heart disease, and may lower the risk of prostate cancer. The recommended daily amount is 30 IU (international units). Synthetic Vitamin E doses up to 1,200 IU per day are generally considered safe, but one recent study questions the safety of taking high-dose daily supplements. Vitamin E should be taken with a meal containing fat so that it can be absorbed properly. Vitamin E is found naturally in vegetable oils, salad dressings and margarines made with vegetable oils, wheat germ, leafy green vegetables, whole grains, and nuts.

Antioxidant

substance that helps reduce damage that can cause cancer or accelerate the aging process. Antioxidants include Vitamins C and E, beta-carotene, flavonoids, and lycopene.

Contrary to popular belief, Vitamin E does not prevent wrinkles or slow other aging processes. Many women report having fewer hot flashes while taking vitamin E, but research study results vary. However, unlike other oils, Vitamin E oil, applied to the vaginal tissue, may be helpful in lubricating the vagina without damaging delicate tissue. While there is no evidence that Vitamin E (up to 700 IU) interferes with blood clotting, some surgeons still recommend stopping Vitamin E supplements prior to surgery.

Whether you are in perimenopause or postmenopause, you should take a multivitamin and mineral supplement daily, especially if you are trying to lose weight. Daily vitamin tablets that are made specifically for postmenopausal women usually do not have iron, but do have more calcium and Vitamin D to help prevent osteoporosis, and extra Vitamins C and E to prevent cell damage and assist the immune system. They also have more of the B vitamins for healthy skin, to assist the body in converting food into energy, and to support the heart, bones, and nervous system. If you have a balanced diet with enough protein, you will not need iron supplements. If you have stopped having periods, you should probably not take vitamins with iron or iron supplements, as the extra iron can build up and cause problems with your blood, spleen, liver, and heart. If you are still getting periods, you should be getting 18 mg of iron per day. If you no longer menstruate, then 8 mg of iron a day is enough. Iron is available in several foods such as poultry, red meat, fruits, eggs, green vegetables, and fortified grain and bread products. Although some studies suggest that taking extra antioxidants or fish oil might help prevent heart disease, results are conflicting, and there are no clear guidelines at present.

Extra folate (folic acid) has long been recommended for pregnant women to prevent birth defects in unborn babies. Some studies suggest that folic acid also lowers the risk of colon and cervical cancer and, in women who drink more than one or two alcohol drinks a day, reduces the risk of breast cancer. Folic acid and the B vitamins are also important for heart and bone health because they decrease a substance in the blood called homocysteine. High levels of homocysteine are linked with heart attacks, Alzheimer's disease, depression, and bones that break more easily. Folic acid is found in green leafy vegetables, orange juice, and fortified cereals.

Getting 400 to 800 IU of Vitamin D daily is important in lowering the risk of bone loss and tooth loss, and also helps decrease falls because it helps with balance. The best food sources of Vitamin D are milk, vitamin-fortified cereals, and fatty fish such as herring and mackerel. Your body can make Vitamin D from sunlight, but it's hard to tell how much sunshine on what amount of exposed skin (unclothed and without sunscreen) is needed to give you enough Vitamin D. So, it's best to rely on food sources and supplements to get your recommended daily amount.

Serotonin

a brain substance associated with good mood and sleep. Some antidepressants (selective serotonin reuptake inhibitors) aid in increasing levels of serotonin.

The B vitamins have many advantages for the menopausal woman. B vitamins help with making red blood cells and **serotonin**, a substance in the body that helps maintain mood. The B vitamins also help to maintain healthy skin, hair, and muscle, and are therefore especially beneficial for menopausal women who often experience dry skin and hair. The B vitamins are present in a wide variety of foods such as fish, poultry, meat, milk, cheese, yogurt, soymilk, watermelons, and whole, fortified, and enriched grains.

Vitamin C is particularly important for healing skin, blood vessels, and making serotonin. It is an antioxidant and assists the immune system. The daily requirement is 75 mg, but you should not exceed 2,000 mg per day if you supplement your intake from food sources. You might reduce your risk for cataracts by taking 500 mg per day. You need to increase your Vitamin C intake if you smoke, if you are regularly exposed to smoke, or if you drink alcohol. You can get plenty of Vitamin C from food sources like citrus fruits, potatoes, broccoli, bell peppers, spinach, strawberries, and tomatoes.

Vitamin A, another antioxidant, is also very important for menopausal women. Women who take more Vitamin A may be less likely to get breast cancer. While normal amounts of Vitamin A are helpful to your eyes (reduces night blindness and preserves normal vision), skin, and bones, excessive intake of Vitamin A can actually be harmful to bones and may increase your risk for a broken bone. The upper limit of Vitamin A is 10,000 IU per day. Vitamin A in the form of **retinoids** is found in beef, eggs, shrimp, fish, milk, and certain kinds of cheeses. Vitamin A in the form of beta carotene is found in the "orange" vegetables like sweet potatoes, carrots, pumpkins, and squash. Spinach, mangos, and turnip greens also contain Vitamin A.

Retinoids

a form of Vitamin A found in beef, eggs, shrimp, fish, milk, and certain kinds of cheeses.

Boron, manganese, phosphorus, zinc, and copper are essential minerals, particularly at midlife. Zinc is needed for the immune system, wound healing, and appears to slow age-related eye disease. Copper assists with red blood cell development. Phosphorus, boron, and manganese help with bone development. Bone pain can be associated with low levels of phosphorus, often caused by poor eating habits or taking too many antacids that bind to phosphorus.

Shana's comment:

Well, one thing I did, when I first started with menopause and the hot flashes, I read that Vitamin E was very good, so I started taking vitamin E. And then I was taking one in the morning and one at night. I think I probably had eight hundred, but then I read somewhere that it was better to take it at night so I started taking two at night before I went to bed. I do think it has helped. I sleep better and maybe that is because I take it at night, I don't really know. But I do know I'm getting sleep.

60. I'm trying to get some relief from my symptoms without having to take estrogen, but when I look at the products that say they will relieve my symptoms, I get very confused. What should I be looking for when I go to the store?

It's most important to carefully read the ingredients.

Inactive ingredient

a filler or sometimes preservative used in the making of some medications and supplements. Although not intended to have any effect on the body, inactive ingredients can sometimes cause reactions.

Tincture

an alcohol-based liquid preparation used for some herbs.

Extract

a concentrated form of a substance, e.g., an herb.

It's most important to carefully read the ingredients. Many herbal products intended for the treatment of menopausal symptoms have multiple herbs in one product, so it's important to know exactly what you would be taking. The primary ingredient in many remedies for menopause symptoms is black cohosh, but other substances can be included in the tablet or capsule. Although there are federal regulations for herbal preparations and dietary supplements, they are not the same as the regulations for prescription medicines, and are often not well enforced. Doses in individual products can vary by hundreds of milligrams. The "filler," additives, or **inactive ingredients** in the preparation may or may not be listed on the label. The label may advertise benefits that have not been proven, and may not have even been studied.

Herbs come in several forms, like **tinctures**, **extracts**, and powders. Tinctures, extracts, and powders contain different herb strengths. The number of milligrams in a tincture is not equivalent to the milligrams in an extract. Also, the different forms may work differently in your body, meaning that a tincture may not work the same way as a ground powder.

In conducting medical research, scientists have found something called the "placebo" effect, meaning that even if the people in the study take nothing more than a sugar pill, 30 to 40% of them will experience some benefit. This placebo effect usually fades over time. That is why long-term studies of medications are so important. The study must continue for a long enough period of time for the initial placebo effect to fade and the true effect of the medication can be evaluated. If the medication really makes a difference, the benefits from the medication will be still be present after the placebo effect has faded. If you take something to relieve your symptoms, you may experience the placebo effect at first. It can take several weeks for both prescription and nonprescription medicines to work. If you have a bad effect from taking something, you should stop taking it and discuss it with your clinician. The main ingredient may not be the problem. Some people can have reactions to inactive ingredients (fillers, preservatives). Sometimes bad effects will fade over time, too. So if your clinician agrees, and the side effects aren't too bad, it might be reasonable to see how it goes for a while. Some products have ingredients like caffeine that can actually make your symptoms worse.

The claims made on some products may not be scientifically based. That doesn't mean that the products will be harmful to you or that you won't benefit from the product in some way. But you need to remember that the FDA does not safeguard against claims made by herb and dietary supplement makers. Look into them carefully on your own before you decide to try one—read about the product on the Internet, talk about it with friends and with your clinician, and then read all of the information on the package carefully before you decide to try it. Always use the lowest possible dose. The FDA says prescriptions should be given in the lowest possible dose that is effective. It makes sense to apply this principle to nonprescription medicines, herbs, and dietary supplements as well.

It's also possible to buy products that contain hormones without a prescription. For example, you can buy progesterone creams at natural food stores and **compounding pharmacies**. Even though these creams have hormones in them, they are sold as dietary supplements or herb products, so they are not evaluated by the FDA in the same way as prescription medications. Independent laboratories have tested products that are sold without prescription (not just those claiming to treat menopause symptoms) and have found that some products contain different amounts than what is listed on the label, or contain ingredients that are not listed. Sometimes these ingredients are not healthy for you. The Consumer Labs web site (*http://consumerlabs.com*) is useful for evaluating herbs. You need to be your own advocate; remember, web sites that sell products are in the business of convincing you to buy their product, and not necessarily in the business of protecting your best interests.

Compounding pharmacies

a pharmacy that specializes in preparing medications (oral, suppositories, creams, tinctures, etc.) that are put together in specific percentages by the compounding pharmacist as prescribed by a clinician. Many compounding pharmacies also carry brand name medications as well.

61. Is there a special "menopause diet"? What foods will help me stay healthy at midlife? Would adding soy products to my diet help my symptoms? Are there specific dietary changes that will ease my hot flashes?

There is no special diet for menopause. Instead, you should eat a healthy balance of complex carbohydrates,

Table 1	The new healthy eating pyramid
Type of food	**Healthy eating recommendations (per day)**
Fats & sweets	• Use olive, soy, corn, sunflower, or peanut oils • Limit saturated fats and trans ("hydrogenated") fats • Limit sweets
Dairy products	• 1–2 servings of low-fat dairy products, a daily calcium supplement, or both
Meat, poultry, fish, eggs, nuts, & legumes	• 1–3 servings of nuts and legumes • 0–2 servings of fish, poultry, or eggs • Choose vegetable sources of protein, such as nuts and beans, more often than animal sources, such as red meat and dairy products
Vegetables & fruits	• 5 or more servings of vegetables • 2–3 servings of fruit
Bread, cereal, & rice	• Eat whole grains and whole-grain products liberally • Limit potatoes and refined carbohydrates such as white bread, white rice, and white potatoes
Multivitamin	• Take one a day

Figure 14   Healthy eating pyramid. Excerpted from *The Benefits and Risks of Vitamins and Minerals Special Health Report.* **© 2003 President and Fellows of Harvard College; reprinted by permission.**

protein, and fats. Figure 14 shows a set of healthy eating guidelines for meats, fruits, vegetables, dairy products, and grains, in addition to recommendations for exercise, alcohol intake, and vitamins. The United States Department of Agriculture and the Department of Health and Human Services intend to release a new, revised food pyramid in early 2005, which will be available on a government web site devoted to nutrition (*www.nutrition.gov*).

Calcium may have additional benefits besides preventing bone loss. Calcium helps with weight loss, reduces the risk of colon cancer, lowers blood pressure, and in men, reduces the risk for prostate cancer. Taking calcium and Vitamin D can help prevent tooth decay as

Eat a healthy balance of complex carbohydrates, protein, and fats.

well. And, calcium taken together with magnesium has been found to reduce PMS (premenstrual symptoms), headaches, and menopausal hot flashes. You can take more magnesium when it is with calcium because it binds with the calcium and will not all be absorbed. Contrary to popular belief, getting the recommended daily amount of calcium up to 1,500 mg does not increase your chances for kidney stones. In fact, getting enough calcium can actually help prevent getting that first kidney stone! If you have already had a kidney stone that has calcium in it, the recommendations for calcium may be different.

Products containing soy are permitted by the FDA to make the claim that getting soy daily reduces the risk of heart disease. The effect of soy on breast tissue is not so straightforward. Because soy contains phyto-estrogens that have some estrogen-like effects, some clinicians have concerns that taking soy may increase the risk of breast cancer. Others point to the low rates of breast cancer in Japanese women who traditionally eat a lot of soy (see Questions 55 and 61 about phytoestrogens and soy). Research results are conflicting as well. However, soy is a good source of protein and contains less fat than animal protein.

Mediterranean diet

a diet high in whole grains, vegetables, tomatoes, olive oil, and moderate amounts of red wine.

Monounsaturated fats

fats derived from plants that are considered healthier than saturated fats from animal sources. Olive oil and safflower oil are examples.

In addition to the healthy eating pyramid (Figure 14), the **Mediterranean diet** is worthy of mention. Although many countries border the Mediterranean Sea, the people of southern Italy and Greece have been well studied because of their lower incidence of heart disease in spite of their higher consumption of fats. However, fat derived from olive oil, which is used freely in their cooking, is **monounsaturated** and does not raise blood cholesterol levels like saturated oils can. The Mediterranean diet recommends red meat no more than once or twice per month. Fish should be eaten regularly, at least once or twice weekly. Choose low-fat dairy products. Eat whole grains, pasta, and crusty breads sparingly. Olive oil and garlic are recommended for cooking. Six to eight ounces of red wine is recommended with the dinner meal because of the antioxidant effect of the red wine. Wine may, however, increase your hot flashes. Lycopene, an antioxidant that is released when tomatoes are cooked, has shown some promise of lowering the risk of prostate cancer, breast and cervical cancer, and heart disease. It's also believed that the lower rate of stomach cancers in Italians is related to their high consumption of tomatoes. The Mediterranean diet also encourages the consumption of berries, legumes such as beans, and nuts such as walnuts and almonds. Berries, particularly blueberries, also contain antioxidants. These help prevent damage that speeds the aging process, and increases your risk for cancer and heart disease.

Making healthy choices is an important part of maintaining a BMI below 25. In addition, there are some basic principles of eating that will help you stay at a healthy weight, which will decrease your symptoms as well:

• Drink water. Six to eight glasses of water (8 oz. each) are recommended each day, in addition to any other beverages you drink. Water helps you stay hydrated, and fills you up without adding extra calories.
• Pay close attention to serving size. For example, a serving size of protein (usually 3 oz.) should be no

larger than the size of a deck of playing cards or the palm of your hand.

- If you add soy to your diet, remember that it has calories, too, and you will need to reduce your calories from other foods in order to add soy.
- Alcohol also has calories. A 6 oz. glass of wine (either white or red) generally has about 130 calories. Drinking more than one glass of wine, one can of beer, or one mixed drink daily can increase your risk of breast cancer.
- Eat the complex carbohydrates found in whole grain foods. Avoid refined sugars such as those found in cakes, cookies, and white bread.
- Avoid saturated fats (animal fat such as ham, steak, butter, and cheese). Peanut butter is high in saturated fat, even though it's derived from a plant. Use monounsaturated fats such as olive oil or safflower oil for cooking, baking, and as salad dressing, rather than vegetable, corn, or peanut oil.
- There are ways that you add calories to your diet, sometimes without realizing it. Avoid tasting food as you cook. Don't eat in front of the television or out of a container. You may be distracted from how much you're eating, and eat more than you realize.
- Increase the fiber in your diet. Higher fiber consumption has been associated with a lower risk of colon cancer, hemorrhoids, constipation, heart disease, and possibly diabetes and other cancers. Fiber is found in grains, fruits, vegetables, nuts, and legumes.
- Limit salt intake to 1,500 mg/day to keep your blood pressure at a normal level. If you read nutrition labels, you might be shocked to learn that one-half cup serving of canned corn contains 360 mg of sodium. Choose foods that are labeled low in sodium or "heart smart."

- Eat foods as close to their natural state as possible. For example, eat an apple, not apple juice, or eat fresh or frozen vegetables rather than canned. Cooking and processing foods often reduces their vitamin and nutrient content, and salt is often used as a preservative in prepared foods.
- It takes the brain about 15 minutes to make you feel full once your stomach is full. Eat slowly so that your brain can register that you've eaten enough before you have seconds or head to the dessert table.
- Get enough calcium in your diet. There is an easy way to figure out how much calcium you are getting: Multiply the number of dairy servings by 250 (you can't count ice cream—it only has 6% of your daily calcium requirement!), and then add 350. So, for example, if you had two glasses of milk (500 mg) and added 350 for the calcium in other foods, you would have consumed 850 mg of elemental calcium. You need enough additional elemental calcium from supplements to give you the recommended 1,300 to 1,500 mg of elemental calcium. That means you'd need an additional 450 to 650 mg of elemental calcium from supplements.
- Exercise daily!

The important thing is to eat a variety of foods so that you get all of the nutrients you need. There are some specific dietary ways that you may be able to reduce your hot flashes:

- Avoid caffeine. This includes coffee, or any caffeine-containing food or beverage such as tea, chocolate milk, and soda. Decaffeinated coffee and hot liquids without caffeine are generally tolerated well. The caffeine rush seems to bring on hot flashes. Even sipping hot cocoa in the coldest weather can bring on a hot flash because the chocolate contains caffeine.

- Avoid refined sugars. The metabolism of simple carbohydrates can increase body fat and increase hot flashes. Despite the recent reports about antioxidant effects in dark chocolate and its ability to stimulate the "good feeling" **endorphins**, chocolates, unfortunately, are best avoided as they are often a double whammy because they contain both refined sugars and caffeine!

- Avoid alcohol. Alcohol increases your skin's temperature, making hot flashes more severe. However, a glass of red wine, though thought to increase hot flashes, can be helpful in reducing your risk of heart disease.

- Eat spicy foods with caution. Some women find that spicy foods can bring on hot flashes.

- Drink more water. Although this won't decrease the incidence of hot flashes for you, keeping well hydrated makes the flashes associated with a lot of sweating much more bearable.

- Consider adding soy. Although research results are conflicting, many women find that soy helps with their hot flashes. Soy is a very healthy food that provides low fat protein, so it's certainly not harmful to include it in your diet. If you find that 20 to 60 grams of soy per day (the recommended daily amount) decreases your hot flashes, so much the better!

- Calcium and magnesium taken together can reduce your hot flashes. The usual dose is 1,000 mg of calcium, with 400 to 500 mg of magnesium.

Each woman will respond differently to different foods and beverages. Keep track of what you eat and

Endorphins

brain chemicals responsible for reducing pain and affecting emotions.

see if it makes a difference, for better or worse, on your hot flashes.

Bridget's comment:

I've learned a lot about trade-offs. I know that one cup of coffee, one beer, or one chocolate bar equals at least eight or nine intense hot flashes. I'll give up the beer and chocolate, but not the coffee. Talking about decisions, maybe I'm paying a price for choosing not to have kids. I missed the pain of labor, but my body has figured out how to deliver a strong dose of the discomfort. Hot flashes take over the same way contractions do. They come in waves, gather and peak, and leave you wiped out and incredulous.

62. How can I manage the stress I've been feeling?

Stress management is very important for women who are having perimenopausal and postmenopausal symptoms because stress can increase your symptoms. Stress can contribute to poor sleep, which can contribute to poor functioning and coping, which can add to your stress. When stress is out of control, symptoms such as hot flashes, forgetfulness, irritability, and lower **libido** get worse. And, when symptoms seem to get out of control, stress can become overwhelming.

Libido
sex drive.

You've probably heard about ways to manage stress since you were young. Figuring out what stresses you and managing those stressors can take years. If lots of things are stressing you out, you will want to start small and concentrate on one stressor at a time.

While it may sound trite, your efforts to resolve stress should be specifically directed at an individual stressor.

For example, if decreased memory or mental function on the job is stressing you, try to identify what is causing the memory and mental performance problems. If lack of sleep is related, then addressing your sleep patterns and minimizing sleep interruptions is important as well (see Question 65 about sleep).

You must make it a priority to find some "down" time. Our society is fast-paced, and the demands to keep up with the pace increase daily. You get up early, you help with family, you go to work, you barely sit for dinner, and when you go to bed, you're faced with hot flashes, night sweats, and thoughts about your day or how you will manage the next day. You get up the next morning, unrested, and start all over again. Who wouldn't be stressed? Somewhere in your busy days, you must find time for yourself:

- *Exercise.* Take a walk. Take a **yoga** class with other stressed women in midlife. Yoga and **tai chi** can both be modified to reduce the risk of vertebral fractures and are very good forms of exercise and relaxation.
- *Share.* You will feel less alone if you share what's going on in your life with other women. Many women feel like no one else suffers with the symptoms of menopause. Talking with other women who do can help you see that you are totally normal, and just knowing that can help reduce your stress.
- *Take a long bath.* Water "therapy" can be very calming. Bubble baths can be irritating to the vulvovaginal area, so don't make it a perfumed bath. Make the time for a 15-minute soak in the tub. Unfortunately, some women do report having hot flashes after showers or baths. Try not to think about all the

Somewhere in your busy days, you must find time for yourself.

Yoga

a form of exercise that combines meditation and flexibility training.

Tai chi

a form of exercise that combines meditation and flexibility training.

things that you have to do while you're soaking! Or, if you really can't get your mind off it, make a list and prioritize so you know what to tackle first.

- *Try redefining your "reward" system.* In place of that candy bar, reward yourself with a slice of free time to get a manicure, massage, or read a novel.

- *Breathe.* **Paced breathing** can be a great way to reduce your stress and become more relaxed. Take a cleansing breath to calm yourself. Breathe in through your nose for a count of 4, hold it for a count of 7, and breathe out for a count of 8. This is particularly good when hot flashes occur at inconvenient or stressful times. Paced breathing has also been shown to help reduce hot flashes, whether it works by decreasing stress that can cause hot flashes or through another biofeedback mechanism is unknown, but, really, who cares—as long as it works!

Paced breathing

a method of breathing used for relaxation. Breathe in for 4 counts, hold for 7 counts, breathe out for 8 counts.

- *Sleep well.* While it may seem obvious to state, make sure that you get a good night's sleep. Good **sleep hygiene** (see Question 65 about sleep hygiene) is critical to sleeping well, and also to stress management. Getting adequate sleep can be the difference between having a stressful day or not. Managing sleep is an underappreciated part of stress management and coping skills.

Sleep hygiene

a group of healthy practices that contribute to a good night's sleep.

- *Progressive relaxation.* Relaxation is often elusive, so you may need to teach yourself how to relax. Start with lying down in a comfortable position, and then gradually tense and relax your muscles. Begin with your feet and legs, move up to your hips, buttocks, and back, then your torso and arms, and finally your face and head. Tense the muscles in each area and then relax them fully. In this way, you teach yourself to feel the relaxed muscles, and

Progressive relaxation

a way to relax by tensing and releasing muscles one at a time.

because you focus your mind on the exercise, you can relax not only tense muscles, but also clear your mind of worrisome thoughts.

- *Laugh.* Laughter is indeed good medicine for stress. Laughter releases endorphins, which are partially responsible for putting you into a good mood. In one study, laughter and humor were found to be important for stress management and were tied to coping better with hot flashes.

There are ways to retrain your reaction to stressful situations so that you can decrease the stress in your life. Sometimes called **coping skills training**, you can learn new ways to solve problems usefully by learning how to analyze a problem, identify possible solutions, decide how to reach the solution you prefer, and make it happen. These skills help you see problems from an objective standpoint, and to change the way you react to the stressor. Your local adult community education program may offer coping skills training, and some HMOs also offer a version of coping skills training that helps with managing migraines and other stress-related illnesses.

Coping skills training

learning new ways to solve problems usefully by learning how to analyze a problem, identify possible solutions, decide how to reach the solution, and make it happen.

Some women drink a glass of wine to help them unwind and relax. A small amount of alcohol is considered part of a healthy diet. But using it to manage stress can backfire. Alcohol can increase hot flashes and cause sleep disruption, even after only one or two glasses of wine. So, it could actually make stress worse. But if a glass of wine really helps you relax, and there is no reason that you should avoid alcohol, then go ahead and enjoy it.

Think about the stressors that are affecting your ability to cope. Then ask yourself what you need to do to change the problem, or the way you react to it. Figure out what you can do realistically to make the changes. Start with one small thing and then add to it over time; don't allow your stress-reduction program to add more stress!

63. I had my children relatively late in life. I have also reached menopause. I'm taking care of young children as well as my parents who are 85 and require a lot of my attention. I'm definitely suffering from caregiver stress while I'm trying to deal with my own aging and menopausal symptoms. How can I manage this particular stress better?

You are not alone in being stressed with caring for aging parents. Approximately 25% of American families are caring for an older adult, an adult child with disabilities, or a sick friend.

The stress of caregiving can be enormous for women sandwiched between caring for children and caring for their parents. The frustration and stress from caring for children and parents can lead to depression, fatigue, anxiety, and illness, all of which can compound your menopausal symptoms. It's important to get some relief from the stress you are experiencing. You might be spending about one third of your life in post-menopause, so it's critical for you to find ways to cope with the stressors of mid and later life, of which care-giving is only one. Search out community programs that might benefit your parents and give you a break. The National Family Caregiver Support Program is a federally funded program that may help you provide care for your parents under the Older Americans Act. (See Question 100 for more resources.)

Stress from caregiving was once thought to actually contribute to the development of breast cancer. But a recent study showed that women who had a high level of stress while caring for a sick, disabled, or elderly family member actually had a lower rate of breast cancer and lower levels of estrogen.

64. Would therapies such as acupuncture, yoga, and massage help my symptoms?

Acupuncture studies show mixed results when it comes to using it for hot flashes. Acupuncture is the practice of inserting needles along the body's meridians (lines) through which qi (pronounced "chi," meaning energy) flows. Acupuncture can be effective for back pain, nausea and vomiting with pregnancy, pain after dental procedures, addiction, arthritis, and headache. There isn't, however, clear evidence that acupuncture will help your menopausal symptoms.

Yoga is a form of exercise, and exercise is important to your health and well being. Engaging in yoga is not harmful, although women with osteoporosis should avoid toe touches due to the risk of spine fractures. It's not clear if yoga, by itself, decreases hot flashes. Exercise has been shown to decrease hot flashes, possibly by reducing stress, and massage may help with hot flashes in a similar way. Using relaxation techniques to reduce hot flashes has also been studied, and the results are promising, particularly when paced breathing is used, and especially when you feel a hot flash starting.

65. What would help me sleep better?

It's important to establish patterns for sleep: going to bed around the same time, waking up around the same time, doing things that your body will get accustomed to doing so that you have good sleep, and eliminating the things that can cause you to stay awake or have periods of waking up.

It's tempting to try to "catch up" on sleep, particularly on the weekends. But when you sleep longer on the weekends, you are undermining your body's ability to fall asleep at the same time in the evening. Establishing and maintaining regular times for going to sleep and waking is important for developing good sleep patterns. This is a big problem for those who have shift work, or who may alternate working days and nights.

When you brush your teeth, put on your pajamas, apply lotion, or do a relaxing activity before bed, you are giving your body and mind the cues that it's time for sleep. Doing the same thing each time you need to fall asleep is important for what is called good sleep hygiene. It's the same idea that's put into practice for young children—developing a quiet routine just before bed helps your mind relax and allows the portion of your brain that controls sleep to take over.

While exercise is extremely important for good health, good bones, stress management, and good sleep, you should not exercise right before going to bed. Sometimes eating right before bed or too far from bedtime can cause problems, causing either digestive upset or a rumbling stomach from hunger pangs. A small snack of protein and carbohydrates right before bed has been shown to chemically make your body and brain more

When you sleep longer on the weekends, you are undermining your body's ability to fall asleep at the same time in the evening.

conducive to sleep. Cottage cheese and crackers, or a container of yogurt sprinkled with soy nuts make for good pre-bedtime snacks.

Developing a good sleep routine also includes limiting your bedroom to sleep and intimate activities. Watching TV, doing work, reading a fast paced murder mystery, doing crossword puzzles, or letting the kids horse around on the bed all contribute to miscues for the body because these activities can stimulate active brain activity. So, even when you think you are ready to sleep, your body has not received the necessary cues.

It's important to eliminate caffeine, alcohol, and nicotine before bed because they can make it difficult to get to sleep and also cause wakenings during the night. Effects from caffeine can bother you for up to 20 hours. Eliminating caffeine may not only help relieve hot flashes that interrupt sleep, but may also allow you to fall asleep more easily. Caffeine and other stimulants are found not only in coffee, tea, and carbonated beverages, but also in chocolate and many cold, allergy, pain, and diet medications. Although alcohol may make you sleepy at first, it may later cause periods of wakefulness through the night. Smoking right before trying to go to sleep also acts as a stimulant instead of calming you down. Other stimulants can interfere with sleep, too, like those found in foods containing monosodium glutamate.

If you are unable get to sleep and stay asleep, you might want to try a sleep restriction program. First, identify how many hours you are currently sleeping. Then, pick a time that you want to get up every day, including weekends, and go to bed so you are in bed only for the amount of time you have been sleeping. So, if you're only able to sleep for a total of 4 hours and you want to get up at 7:00 am, you will start going to bed at 3:00 am. Once you've been able to sleep for the full 4 hours or for 95% of the 4 hours for several nights, go to bed 30 minutes earlier. In a stepwise fashion, after you are consistently sleeping for 95% of the time that you are in bed, again make your bedtime 30 minutes earlier. Continue this pattern until you are sleeping for 7 to 8 hours. You will spoil the program if you use **sedatives**, stimulants (including caffeine and alcohol), or take naps.

Doing relaxing activities such as writing in a journal, having a warm cup of herb tea, or reading a relaxing book (no work-related reading!) can help you get in the mood to sleep. Progressive relaxation techniques (see Question 62 about stress management) and deep breathing can often relax you enough to go to sleep.

If you are waking from hot flashes and night sweats, it's especially important to sleep in a well-ventilated, cool room with a light blanket. To avoid disrupting sleep even more, some women keep a towel next to the bed with an extra nightgown to slip into without having to get out of bed, turn on the light, or change the sheets. There are also pajamas made with material that wicks the sweat away from your body, keeping you more comfortable after night sweats. These wicking pajamas are marketed especially for women who are experiencing hot flashes and night sweats to reduce the discomfort of sweat-drenched pajamas. If you are observing a good sleep routine and are still not getting good sleep, you should talk to your clinician about

Sedative

a medication intended to produce a calming effect.

going on something that will relieve your hot flashes and night sweats.

There are several nonprescription products that are advertised to help you sleep. The active ingredient in most of these products is Benadryl® (diphenhydramine), an **antihistamine** found in many cold and allergy preparations. Benadryl® can cause a hangover effect for some people, especially if you take as much as 50 mg. Antihistamines can also cause drying of the mucous tissues such as your eyes, mouth, and vaginal walls, making some menopausal symptoms worse.

Botanicals such as valerian, passion flower, lemon balm, German chamomile, and lavendar hops can have sedative effects, and are available over the counter, but have not been well studied. **Melatonin**, a pineal gland hormone important for the sleep-wake cycle, has been used to treat jet lag or sleep disturbances in shift workers, but has not been proven to improve sleep onset or decrease night waking. Don't forget the home remedy of a glass of warm milk before bedtime—the substances in the milk that are released when it is warmed can cause drowsiness.

As a last resort, a very short course of a sedative can be prescribed so that you can fall asleep more easily. But whatever you take, it should not become part of your nightly routine for the long term. Instead, the underlying reason for your sleep disturbances should be treated, such as hot flashes, depression, anxiety, or a new medical condition. Prescription sleeping pills can be addictive, and when you stop taking them there is often a rebound effect causing you to have poor sleep once again.

Antihistamine

a medication intended to reduce allergic reactions; also dries mucous membranes such as the mouth and vagina.

Botanicals

any plant, although used mostly in reference to herbs or flowers, that is used medicinally.

Melatonin

a pineal gland hormone important for the sleep-wake cycle and used to treat jet lag or sleep disturbances in shift workers, but has not been proven to improve sleep onset or decrease night waking.

Since there are medical conditions that can cause sleep disturbances, such as asthma or overactive thyroid, it's important to discuss your symptoms with your clinician. Getting medical conditions under control can help you sleep much better, too.

Jackie's comment:

I did have one really bad summer when the weather was hot in Maine and I had the worst of the hot flashes. I've never really been a really good sleeper. I only need 6 or 7 hours a night. I don't take naps but I drink a lot of water and get up almost every night. My philosophy is if I don't sleep long enough one night, I just sleep a little more the next. And I just try to stay positive.

66. Vaginal dryness is a big problem for me. What can I do about it?

Vaginal dryness caused by the low estrogen levels of postmenopause can be extremely uncomfortable, particularly during sexual intercourse. Some women can't sit comfortably because of the vaginal and urinary changes, which include dryness and lack of elasticity around the sensitive tissue of the urethra and vagina.

For vaginal dryness, there are some products that will help lubricate the vaginal walls, particularly during sexual activity. KY Personal Lubricant Jelly®, Astroglide®, Lubrin®, and Moist Again® are examples of nonhormonal, short-acting, water-based lubricants that are safe to use. Should you be uncomfortable at times other than during sex, there are longer-acting moisturizers available, such as Replens® and KY Long-Acting Moisturizer®. Moisturizers, even ones specifically made for vaginal dryness, are not a substitute for lubricants. Never use an oil-based lubricant or moisturizer such as petroleum jelly or hand lotion because they can injure tissue. Petroleum jelly and other oil-based products such as hand cream or baby oil do not absorb well in the vagina, are difficult to remove, can be irritating, and can cause breakdown of condoms or diaphragms. Vitamin E oil, however, is an exception and is considered safe and nonirritating. Perfumed or deodorized products, including lubricants, soaps, feminine hygiene products, and toilet tissue, also can be irritating and may cause infection. Douching will not moisturize the vagina. Instead it dries out the tissue and flushes out the normal flora, changing the normal acidic balance, also increasing risk of infection. Some women try to restore the normal vaginal bacteria with yogurt. Not only is this messy, it doesn't work and may be irritating.

Never use an oil-based lubricant or moisturizer such as petroleum jelly or hand lotion because they can injure tissue.

Hormones that are used throughout the body in the form of pills, creams, patches, gels, or injections, and those applied directly to the vagina, such as creams, rings, or suppositories, will help vaginal dryness. They can be used alone or with vaginal lubricants or moisturizers. Vaginal creams, rings, and suppositories tend to offer relief very quickly while other forms can take longer. (See Question 76 for more information about hormones used vaginally.)

Even if your vaginal dryness does not feel like a problem, it makes you more susceptible to vaginal infection and transmission of sexually transmitted infections (STIs). Using pre-lubricated condoms can be a good option since they provide more protection against STIs and have lubrication already on them. If you are taking antihistamines for allergies, your vaginal dryness may be worse.

Having sex more often may reduce your discomfort. Sex during the postmenopause years is one of those "use it or lose it" situations. Your body will respond to the ongoing stimulation: the more often you have sex, the more lubrication and less dryness you will experience. However, most women do not substantially change their interest in sex following menopause. You are unlikely to suddenly be interested in having sex several times weekly if your usual habit was to have sex once a week or a few times a month. The bottom line is to continue at your own comfortable pace, use lubricants as needed, and allow for more foreplay to maximize your natural lubrication—and remember that sex can continue to be comfortable, satisfying, and enjoyable.

Having sex more often may reduce your discomfort.

67. Will anything help my sex drive? I have heard that DHEA might be helpful.

Your lack of sex drive during perimenopause and postmenopause is not at all uncommon. It's also one of the more complex problems of menopause. Sex drive has as much to do with your brain and emotions as it does with your vagina and your hormones. So, there are no easy solutions.

Female sexual dysfunction (FSD) is a medical condition, and symptoms include lack of desire for sex, lack of arousal during sex, lack of ability to reach orgasm, or pain during intercourse. All of these symptoms can become more apparent and bothersome after menopause. Approximately 43% of all women report some degree of sexual dysfunction.

Female sexual dysfunction (FSD)

a medical condition characterized by symptoms including lack of desire for sex, lack of arousal during sex, lack of ability to reach orgasm, or pain during intercourse.

Before heading for the drug store for a prescription, it's probably a good idea to have a look at reasons why your sex drive might be flagging:

- Is your diminished sex drive related to the physical aspects of perimenopause and menopause?
  - Are your periods irregular, and therefore your hormone levels erratic?
  - Are you experiencing vaginal dryness? Use water-based lubricants to make sex more comfortable. Talk with your clinician about hormone therapy if using lifestyle and alternative therapies have not worked for you in making sex more comfortable.
  - Fear of getting pregnant can interfere with your sex drive. Using reliable birth control during perimenopause can help you relax.
  - Are you feeling overly stressed or too tired for sex? Perimenopause and early postmenopause are often times of newly diagnosed depression. You may need a checkup for that fatigue you've been experiencing. Lack of interest in sex can be a result of fatigue, which can be a result of poor sleep and stress. You may also be overwhelmed by work, family troubles, or health concerns.
- Are you on medications that can affect your sexual function? Some medicines for depression and high blood pressure can make you less physically responsive and make it difficult to have an orgasm.
- Do you have concerns about your body that make you feel unattractive? How you respond to sex during menopause can also be linked to your body image. You may not be comfortable with weight you've gained or skin that feels dry. See Question 95 about your body image during menopause. Fear of

being incontinent or leaking urine during sex can also make you avoid intimacy (see Questions 26, 68, and 90 about urinary incontinence).

- Have you made some effort around changing your sexual routine with your partner, such as having sex in different places, using different sexual positions, making dates, going on vacations devoted to sex, using a finger-tip personal massager or vibrator, reading or watching erotic materials together, using toys or fantasy play? Are you allowing enough time for stimulation? Do you need to reevaluate your relationship with your partner? Are there other issues besides sex that could be affecting your connection with each other? Chances are your partner may be experiencing some midlife changes as well. Menopause is a good time to rekindle your relationships or reevaluate their place in your life.

Because your **clitoris** will have decreased blood flow as you age, it will become less sensitive, and it may become more difficult for you to become aroused. Sexual response and enjoyment can also be diminished because sensation in the clitoris decreases with lower estrogen levels. The less aroused you are, the more difficult it is to become lubricated. A decrease in lubrication is to be expected during postmenopause as well, but using vaginal lubricants and moisturizers can keep the vagina from being too dry and unreceptive to penetration (see Question 66 about vaginal dryness). There are also some ways to increase blood flow to the clitoris and genitals:

Clitoris

female counterpart of the penis that becomes erect with sexual stimulation. Unlike the penis, the clitoris does not house the urethra. The clitoris is located just in front of the urethral opening under a "hood" of tissue and is sensitive to stimulation. See Figure 8, page 45.

- Take a warm bath. The warm water will increase blood flow to the area by dilating blood vessels.

- Take more time for foreplay. The longer you work on getting aroused, the better the blood flow and lubrication, and thus sensation and enjoyment.
- Try using a cream or oil preparation that contains **L-arginine**. Several different products are available such as Alura™, Femore™, and Vigel™. L-arginine is known to increase blood flow to the genitals when taken by mouth, but research has not been conducted that proves that this is true when applied right to the genitals in a cream, so results may vary. Use caution if you have had herpes because L-arginine can increase herpes outbreaks. Most of these products are made with menthol-based creams or oils. Menthol will cause some tingling and warmth where it is applied, and may enhance sensation. But menthol can be irritating and drying as well, so be cautious if you decide to try these. If the sensation from menthol is pleasant, some people advise that a partner suck on a menthol lozenge or breath mint prior to or during oral sex. Do not use menthol creams intended for relieving sore muscles.
- Trial a clitoral suction device. Clitoral suction devices have a small suction cup that is applied to the clitoris, and a gentle suction pump is used to bring blood flow to the area. The suction increases sensation, lubrication, and the ability to have an orgasm. The only FDA-approved clitoral suction device is Eros-Therapy™ made by Urometrics and available only with a prescription. Less costly versions of suction devices have not been well studied.

L-arginine

a substance known to increase blood flow to the clitoris.

DHEA (dehydro-epiandrosterone)

a steroid that has androgen effects.

DHEA (dehydroepiandrosterone) is a steroid that has androgen effects. It is made mostly in the adrenal glands, and a small portion in the ovaries. DHEA in the body reaches peak levels when women are in their mid-20s and falls off almost completely by the time they are 70 years of age. DHEA made from wild yam and soy is getting a lot of attention because of its claims to slow down the aging process and, in particular, improve sex drive.

The varying amounts of DHEA in creams and oral preparations make it difficult to prescribe a particular amount or to know how much will be absorbed. DHEA has been advertised as helpful to memory and energy. Some studies show it helps with energy and sex drive, but others showed no improvement in memory. There are women who report that DHEA is helpful in improving memory, muscle, energy, and sex drive.

Oral doses around 50 mg or less do not appear to have bad side effects in older patients. But since DHEA is a steroid with testosterone-related activity, side effects such as facial hair and acne can occur even with lower dosages. High dosages can cause other serious side effects like jaundice, liver problems, depression, changes in cholesterol levels, and male characteristics such as decreased breast tissue, deepened voice, and increased hair growth, or even liver cancer. Talk with your clinician before you take or use DHEA.

DHEA is banned by the International Olympic Committee because it is a precursor to testosterone, which is also banned. DHEA has also been banned in Canada because safety information is not available.

A few other products are also marketed for treatment of sexual dysfunction, such as Avlimil®, Cerniplex®, ArginMax®, and Zestra®. Although it is touted as "100% natural," the main ingredient in Avlimil® is sage, which can have serious effects on the nervous system and can cause side effects like hallucinations or seizures. The ingredients of Cerniplex® are hard to identify because they are advertised as a "blend of Chinese herbs." While some Chinese herb mixtures are very useful, they are usually prepared individually by a Chinese herbalist in a mixture that is specifically formulated for an individual woman's problems and body chemistry.

ArginMax® and Zestra®, however, may offer some hope. ArginMax® is an oral product that has L-arginine, damiana, ginseng, and ginko biloba. Clinical trials indicated a significant improvement in sexual function and satisfaction after 4 weeks of treatment. Women who have herpes outbreaks should use Argin-Max® with caution since L-arginine has been associated with increasing the frequency of outbreaks. Zestra® contains a blend of oils such as evening primrose, borage seed, extract of coleus, extract of angelica, and antioxidants, and is massaged into the genitals during foreplay. Women with female sexual dysfunction reported much greater sexual response after use of Zestra®. Effects are usually noticed within about 5 minutes, and last for about 45 minutes. Zestra® was designed for use with foreplay, manual stimulation, masturbation, and vaginal sex, but is not intended for oral sex. As you explore options for increasing your interest in and enjoyment of sex, it is important to remember to practice "safer sex." Unless you have a monogamous relationship with a partner who is also monogamous, you continue to be at risk for sexually transmitted infections, so condoms with **spermicide**, even when pregnancy is not an issue, offer the best protection. If this reminder is dampening your enjoy-

Spermicide

a jelly-type or foam substance used with condoms and diaphragms to kill sperm as a form of birth control. Some types of spermicide also reduce the risk for some sexually transmitted infections.

ment or interest, remember that creatively applying condoms can be part of foreplay.

68. I am struggling with the embarrassment of urinary incontinence. Is there anything I can do to manage this symptom better?

Women with urinary incontinence can feel more than embarrassment. Concerns about having "accidents," odor, and appearance can lead to social isolation and depression. Urinary issues can also cause sexual, physical, mental, social, career, and financial problems. Some women have the mistaken notion that drinking fewer fluids means less incontinence. Restricting fluids really doesn't help incontinence, and can lead instead to dehydration and constipation, and may increase the odor of urine due to its concentration. Women may no longer feel desirable and decline sexual relations with their partners due to odor and discomfort or concerns about leaking. This can lead to relationship problems with a partner or spouse. The stress that women experience because of incontinence can also increase their menopausal symptoms.

Restricting fluids really doesn't help incontinence, and can lead instead to dehydration and constipation.

Most treatments for both urge and stress urinary incontinence start with behavioral approaches. The following bladder retraining program is more successful if you have urge incontinence:

- Keep a voiding diary, writing down each visit to the toilet, the amount of leakage, if anything prompted the leakage (laughing, sneezing, coughing, etc.), or the urge to urinate. The diary will give you an idea of the frequency of your trips to the bathroom, the degree of leakage, and what prompts the urge and leakage.

- Figure out the frequency of your trips to the bathroom, and start making trips more often than you usually urinate or leak; so if you leak every 1½ hours, you'd plan to go to the bathroom once an hour. Go to the bathroom at that frequency and empty your bladder even if you don't have the urge to go.

- Once you have been on your new schedule for 2 full days without an accident, increase the time between scheduled trips to the bathroom by 15 to 30 minutes. Keep adding time in a step-wise manner. Before increasing the time between trips, make sure you have gone 2 days without leakage.

- Bladder retraining can take many weeks. Don't be discouraged if it takes you a few months to get enough control to reduce visits to the bathroom to once every 3 to 4 hours.

- If you get the urge to urinate when you are not in the bathroom, try the following to reduce the urge: stand still, relax, take a big breath, and let it out slowly. What you're trying to do is get control over the urge ("mind over bladder"). Concentrate on the urge, and imagine it's like being in a car going up a mountain and coming down the other side. Once the peak of the urge has gone by, you're on your way down, and the urge to urinate will become less. You can also try distracting activities such as counting backwards, reading something interesting, exhaling slowly, or talking on the phone. While suppressing the urge to go, it's important to stay still and tense your pelvic muscles. You can figure out which muscles to tense by intentionally stopping the flow of urine when you are urinating into the toilet. This will help you locate the right muscles to squeeze when you get the urge to go at an unscheduled or inconvenient time. For women who have normal frequency of trips to the bathroom but have sudden urges, learning "urge suppression" can be really helpful. After gaining control over the urge, walk to the bathroom and empty your bladder.

Exercises for the pelvic muscles, which are used to start and stop the flow of urine, are called **Kegel exercises** and are particularly helpful for women with stress incontinence. However, all women should do Kegels, regardless of whether they are incontinent. The muscles that you exercise doing Kegels are not those in your buttocks, your abdomen, or your thighs. Focus only on the muscles controlling the flow of urine (see Figure 15). Contract these muscles for a count of 5 to 10 seconds. Relax the muscles for a count of 10 seconds. Repeat this until you've worked up to 10 minutes of exercise. But don't start out doing Kegels for 10 minutes—like any muscle, exercising them too much

Kegel exercises

tensing and releasing muscles that surround the urethra and vagina. Kegels are intended to help relieve stress incontinence, and to also strengthen vaginal and pelvic muscles.

All women should do Kegels, regardless of whether they are incontinent.

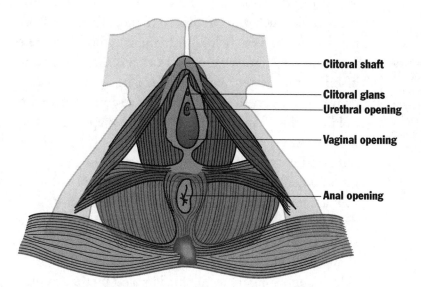

Clitoral shaft

Clitoral glans
Urethral opening

Vaginal opening

Anal opening

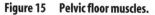

Figure 15   Pelvic floor muscles.

in the beginning can cause pain and too much stress to the muscle. The goal is to build up slowly so that you can exercise your pelvic muscles for 10 minutes, twice a day. The old way of doing Kegels (i.e., quickly tense then relax the pelvic muscles) is not as effective at increasing muscle strength. The results are much better when the exercises are done intentionally, and repeated for a sustained period of time, just as **aerobic exercises** are more effective at improving your heart status when they're done for a sustained period of time.

Special weights held in the vagina can be used to help focus the exercises, and improve muscle strength. Developing stronger muscles has even better results than medicine in treating stress incontinence. Ask your gynecologic clinician about how to order weights—some may be available through your clinician's office. Others can be ordered on the Internet.

A **pessary** is a device that is fitted by an urologist or gynecologist. It goes into the vagina and provides some support between the urethra and the vaginal wall. A pessary can be very helpful for women who have stress incontinence, or uterine or bladder prolapse (when the bladder drops lower into the abdomen). Both can cause extra pressure on the bladder and cause problems with holding urine. Some pessaries look like diaphragms and must be removed periodically for cleaning. If a pessary is not fitted properly, the woman can develop areas of irritation where the pessary rubs on the vaginal tissue. If you are experiencing stress incontinence and vaginal dryness, the vaginal estrogen ring may provide both the estrogen and the support you need. See Appendix B about hormone therapy. Tampons can sometimes provide enough support to the bladder and urethra to prevent urine leakage, but tampons can also dry out the

Aerobic exercise

exercise intended to strengthen your heart, such as running, cycling, or brisk walking, by increasing your breathing and heart rate; this type of exercise helps your body burn off fat and helps control cholesterol.

Pessary

a device that's fitted into the vagina and provides some support between the urethra and the vaginal wall. It is fitted by a urologist or gynecologist, but may be removed, cleaned, and inserted again at home by a woman.

vaginal tissue because they are absorbent. You must remember to change a tampon every 4 to 6 hours to prevent **toxic shock syndrome**.

As part of the behavioral changes you need to make in managing incontinence, it's important to avoid constipation. Straining to eliminate hard stool will damage your pelvic muscles, causing more urinary incontinence. Getting enough water, eating more fiber, and getting regular exercise can help reduce constipation.

There are pads that are specifically designed for urinary incontinence. You should avoid using sanitary pads that are made for menstrual blood because they tend to be very coarse and irritating if used constantly for urine. Menstrual pads are not absorbent enough to capture all the urine, making odor worse, and causing more embarrassment. Since menstrual pads are ineffective, women can end up spending too much money on something that won't hold urine.

Pads made for urinary incontinence are available at your local pharmacy or grocery store, as well as online. Pads come in several sizes and absorbencies. Undergarments meant for urine leakage are also available and come in various sizes just like underwear. Some undergarments come with a waterproof pouch for pads, giving extra protection from leaking through to clothing. Undergarments may be the kind that you can pull on and off like regular underwear, or come with side adhesive or Velcro to make changing them easier. Pads and undergarments come in either disposable or reusable forms. Pads to protect bedding and furniture are all available in disposable or reusable versions as well. Pads and undergarments can be expensive and may not be covered by insurance.

Toxic shock syndrome

a condition characterized by sudden onset of high fever, vomiting, rash, and eventually shock, usually as a result of a blood infection caused by a tampon that has stayed in the vagina too long.

Lifestyle Changes and Alternative Therapies

Even the pads made specifically for incontinence can breed bacteria, making you more susceptible to infection. They should be changed often to prevent skin breakdown. If you develop a fever, have more urgency or frequency, see blood in your urine, smell stronger or foul-smelling urine, or have pain when you urinate, you must contact your clinician to have your urine tested.

Some lifestyle changes will help you manage stress incontinence. The National Institutes of Health recommend the following:

- Regulate your bowels to avoid constipation. Try increasing fiber in your diet.
- Quit smoking to reduce coughing and bladder irritation. Smoking also increases your risk of bladder cancer.
- Avoid alcohol and caffeinated beverages, particularly coffee, which can overstimulate your bladder. (Since alcohol and caffeine can aggravate hot flashes, you would be helping manage two symptoms at one time.)
- Lose weight if you need to (the increased pressure in your belly from extra weight can increase leakage).
- Avoid foods and drinks that may irritate your bladder, such as spicy foods, carbonated beverages, and citrus fruits and juices.
- Keep blood sugars under good control if you have diabetes.
- If you are taking water pills (diuretics) for other health problems, consult your clinician about the timing of your medication.

Although as many as one third of women over the age of 50 may experience some form of incontinence, the actual numbers are not known. Many women are so embarrassed that they are reluctant to speak with their clinicians about it. If you are having any form of incontinence, whether you feel you are managing it well or not, you should discuss it with your clinician who may help you manage it better or refer you to a specialist. See Question 90 about additional medications, surgeries, and urethral inserts for managing incontinence.

Women can become secretive about this problem, leading them into social isolation. They may worry so much about odor or the location of the nearest toilet that they distance themselves from friends or family. It's very important for women to be comfortable confiding in those who can help them with incontinence, and to avoid social isolation and depression.

Sarah's comment:

I've been amazed how easily women my age talk about menopausal changes in regard to sleep, mood swings, and even lack of sexual desire, but NOT about incontinence. It's embarrassing, and they think they're the only one who has the problem or it's because of having 2 or 3 children close together. When talking with anyone about menopause, I always bring the subject up—women need to know that there can be alternatives depending on the diagnostic testing outcomes. I only wish doctors were more open about this subject with their menopausal patients. All that's ever discussed is June Allison's Depends' advertisement and "I gotta go—I gotta go" ad. That's not right. This is as important to women as the need for Viagra is to men.

69. Will regular exercise help my symptoms? What kind of exercise is most appropriate during menopause?

Many women report having fewer hot flashes and better sleep after exercising regularly. Because exercise has been shown to increase the release of endorphins, mood can improve and chronic pain can be lessened by regular exercise. Regular exercise has also been shown to prevent and reduce the risk of developing heart disease, diabetes, obesity, and bone loss.

Your goal should be to exercise 30 minutes every day; however, getting even 30 minutes of exercise several times per week can help reduce your risk of heart disease. Some clinicians say that the 30 minutes should be done all at one time, while others say that 10 minutes of exercise done three different times during the day, like walking to and from your car, each count toward the total of 30 minutes per day. The important thing is to get out, get moving, and be as physically active as you can. Do not, however, start an intensive exercise program without consulting your clinician first. And don't be discouraged if you have hot flashes while exercising. This often happens, so many women who are having menopausal symptoms prefer to do all of their exercise at one time and shower afterward, rather than dividing exercise up throughout the day. The overall benefit of regular exercise far outweighs the inconvenience of having a hot flash or two during exercise when you may already be perspiring!

Exercise should not be limited to physical activity. Exercising your brain is extremely important during postmenopause. Keep your brain engaged and do activities that require focus, concentration, and memory. You should be doing things that are mentally challenging to you, like doing crossword puzzles, having intellectual conversations, developing new hobbies, or following news events—anything that exercises your mind and keeps it active.

Exercising your brain is extremely important during post-menopause.

Aerobic exercise is important for your heart health. Such exercise includes brisk walking, jogging, running, swimming, bicycling, and cross-country skiing, as long as the activity increases your breathing and heart rate. High-intensity conditioning should be approved by your clinician before you start. Some suggest that regular sexual activity is "doubly" good for the heart. Not only does sex increase your heart rate and provide some aerobic activity, it can also be good for your heart emotionally.

You should also exercise to prevent bone loss. It's important to remember that the exercises must be weight bearing and provide resistance to your muscles. (See Question 39.)

Resistive exercises are those where the muscles are pushing and pulling. Lifting weights or using weights during exercise is ideal for exercising to prevent bone loss. Swimming, although not a weight-bearing exercise, is a great option because it's resistive as well as aerobic. Bicycling and walking are not ideal for reducing the risk of bone loss because they do not exercise the upper body. They do, however, provide you with

Resistive exercises
exercises where the muscles must push and pull against force, such as weight training and swimming.

the kind of exercise that may improve sleep and generally make you feel better, and they are excellent aerobic exercises that will help prevent heart disease. You can also combine exercises by carrying hand weights and swinging your arms while walking or running. This will provide both aerobic exercise for your heart and bone strengthening resistance exercises for your legs, spine, and arms.

Tai chi is good exercise for women at risk for bone loss, as is yoga, as long as you avoid forward bending at the waist if you already have osteoporosis (see Question 40 about osteoporosis).

Shana's comment:

I like exercising. When I do exercise and I drink a lot of water, I do feel better. I'm not crying, I don't feel depressed and about those hot flashes, it just keeps them away for a while. It's best if I can do it every day. Sometimes I miss and then I can really tell—the flashes come right back!

70. How should I dress to make hot flashes more bearable?

Dress in layers so that when you start to feel warm, you can remove clothing as needed. Sleeveless shirts under a sweater or jacket may provide you with the professional look without the added warmth from long-sleeved shirts. Always wear breathable fabrics such as cotton, and avoid fabrics that tend to increase sweating, like polyester, silk, and synthetics. Instead, wear clothing that won't show perspiration as much. If you perspire heavily during hot flashes, avoid linen because it tends to show sweat more easily. Select clothing that is made from washable fabrics so you can launder them easily, and to reduce extra costs from dry cleaning. Avoid turtlenecks; instead, consider wearing a scarf or fake turtleneck ("dickie") that you can easily remove if needed, or select open or V-neck shirts.

Nylon slips and nylon stockings may be a particular problem if you experience profuse sweating because they do not absorb sweat well. There are some new synthetic fabrics that wick sweat away from the body, like the material used by runners. This material is good for exercising but is rarely used in everyday clothing, with the exception of pajamas. Some pajamas made from material that wicks sweat are now being advertised for women who experience night sweats.

Wool, although a natural fabric, tends to keep you warmer and is frequently lined with a synthetic fabric like rayon, a combination that could worsen the discomfort of hot flashes and sweats. Sometimes women wear sleeveless shells under wool jackets in the winter to stay more comfortable. It's also helpful to have a spare shirt at work or nightgown and sheets beside your bed to change if needed.

Bridget's comment:

Marinating in all this sweat makes me very irritable. Rashes spring up in creases and folds. I'm always damp and itchy. Forget make-up. It washes off with the first flash of the morning. My hair is limp and scraggly before I'm out the front door. I even sweat between my toes and worry about jungle rot in the dead of winter. My dry cleaning and clothing bills have skyrocketed. Only 100 percent natural breathable fibers offer some relief. In 10-degree mid-February weather with the car window wide open, I must look deranged to fellow drivers. What they don't know is that two or three times an hour, I've got the AC on full blast at the coldest setting with vents aimed straight at my face and neck. I've bought fans for home and office, the kind you unfold and wave in front of your face, but I'm still working up the courage to flick one open in public.

71. How do I manage the assortment of other symptoms I have?

Menopause can also bring a bunch of new symptoms that may feel totally unrelated to one another, such as dry eyes, heart palpitations, headaches, and joint pain. Some women will only get hot flashes. Others will get the entire smorgasbord of symptoms.

Eye lubricants, in the form of gel, ointment, or drops, are helpful for dry eyes. Be aware that some eye drops, depending on their contents, can interact badly with your contact lenses. Ointments should be used before bed because they tend to cause some blurring. In severe cases of dry eye, your eye care professional can discuss surgery to plug up the tear ducts (called punctal plugs) so that tears are redirected to lubricate the eye. Prescription eye drops such as steroid drops that reduce inflammation have also been found to be helpful in the treatment of dry eyes. You can decrease the risk of developing **macular degeneration**, an eye disease that can lead to blindness, by using sunglasses or hats to reduce your exposure to bright sunlight, and taking a multiple vitamin that includes antioxidants, zinc, and lutein. Your eye care professional must evaluate changes in vision.

Macular degeneration

the most common cause of blindness in postmenopausal women. Caused by a deterioration in part of the retina, resulting in a progressive loss of central vision.

Many women experience discomfort with contact lenses in postmenopause. You may need to re-wet them several times per day with an appropriate lubricant, or try lenses with higher water content. You should also remove your contacts for a few hours each day.

Heart palpitations can be downright scary. Many things can cause them: stress, sleep deprivation, stimulants like caffeine, alcohol, cold medicines, monosodium gluta-mate, or nicotine, and health problems like thyroid dis-orders and diabetes. And when the palpitations start, it can raise your stress further, making them worse. You need to get this symptom checked out before you chalk it up to menopause. If it is just menopause, then you can reduce palpitations by avoiding all stimulants (including chocolate!). Exercise can help to get the heart rate stable and may help you feel less anxious, so you might have fewer palpitations to begin with. Stress management techniques like deep breathing can help when palpitations are there, but be careful that you don't overdo it and hyperventilate. You need to pay attention and notice what types of things set off your palpitations, and it might help to write them down in a diary—when palpitations happen, foods, activities, stress, exercise, and so forth. Then look it over to see if there is any type of pattern; the things that set off palpi-tations (triggers) can be different for every person.

Not everyone has the same headache triggers, either. Chocolate, aged cheese, and red wine are common trig-gers, as are too much or too little sleep, skipping meals, and stress. Caffeine may help a headache, but it can also cause headaches. If you have been a big caffeine drinker, withdraw slowly from caffeine by gradually mixing in more and more decaffeinated beverages to prevent withdrawal headaches. Irregular hormone lev-els can cause headaches during menstruation and peri-menopause. Sometimes women get fewer headaches in postmenopause if they have had migraine headaches previously linked with their periods. Some women experience worse headaches in postmenopause if they feel more stressed or if they are on hormone therapy for hot flashes. See Question 62 about reducing and managing stress.

Taking magnesium supplements has been shown to help headaches. You should take calcium with the magnesium. In addition to the recommended daily allowance of 320 mg of magnesium from food sources, you should not take more than 350 mg per day of magnesium as a supplement. Magnesium also helps to soften stool and reduces constipation (it helps the intestines move food through better), improves mood, and when combined with calcium reduces premenstrual symptoms and hot flashes. Acupuncture and magnet therapy have both shown some promise in the treatment of headaches.

Glucosamine
condroitin

a supplement that can help joint pain and arthritis. It provides nutrition to the cartilage around the joints.

Glucosamine condroitin supplements can help joint pain and arthritis. Glucosamine provides nutrition to the cartilage around the joints. It is important to exercise to strengthen bones and muscles so that joints are well supported. If you are overweight, your joints will more than likely become less painful if you lose some weight. Massage therapy has also been helpful in relieving the pain associated with arthritis.

See Table 13, which summarizes some nonprescription strategies for managing your menopausal symptoms.

Table 13 Nonprescription Management of Some Common Menopausal Symptoms

Symptom	Management Suggestions
Decreased sex drive	Sensual massage; warm bath; erotica; fantasy play; use of sex toys; take more time; suction devices; menthol creams intended for vaginal/clitoral use; change sexual routine; DHEA
Dry eyes	Lubricant drops; try different types of contact lenses; wear contact lenses less; remember to blink, particularly when using computers or reading; avoid use of antihistamines
Forgetfulness/ lack of concentration	Keep mind active with puzzles, intellectual pursuits, and hobbies; use timers, alarms, and lists for remembering; get adequate sleep
Headaches	Magnesium supplements; biofeedback; acupuncture; avoid food triggers and alcohol; get adequate sleep (not too much or too little); use stress management techniques
Heart palpitations	Paced respirations; avoid caffeine, alcohol, cold preparations such as Sudafed; use stress management techniques
Hot flashes	Avoid caffeine, alcohol, nicotine, spicy foods; drink 6 to 8 glasses of water/day; Vitamin E; increase calcium and magnesium; stop smoking; wear layered clothes of breathable fabrics; paced respirations; increase soy in diet; exercise regularly; acupuncture; black cohosh and other herbs
Joint pain	Massage; whirlpool baths; exercise; lose weight; glucosamine condroitin supplements
Night sweats	Use a fan; keep room cool; sleep in cotton or wicking fabric pajamas; all of the above for hot flashes
Sleeplessness	Reduce hot flashes with strategies listed above; have a carbohydrate and protein snack, or a cup of warm milk; develop good sleep routines; have partner or self evaluated for snoring; don't eat or drink close to bedtime; don't exercise before bed (except for sex); valerian and passion flower herbs
Stress/irritability	Focus on fixing one specific stressor at a time; massage; paced breathing; take a vacation, if only in your head; exercise; progressive relaxation; healthy diet; decrease alcohol; leisurely bath; develop a better sleep routine; share your menopause experiences with other women; find time for laughter; get relief from hot flashes and night sweats
Urinary incontinence	Kegel exercises; "train" bladder; avoid alcohol and caffeine; wear pessary or tampon vaginally; try urethral inserts especially during exercise
Vaginal dryness	Water-based lubricants; vaginal moisturizers; alternative forms of sex (oral, mutual masturbation); decrease use of antihistamines; increase frequency of intercourse

72. As a breast cancer survivor, I've been told that I can't have hormone therapy to treat my hot flashes and other symptoms of menopause. What will help me?

Breast cancers can either be estrogen-receptor positive or not, or someplace in between, meaning that the cancer can be strongly linked to estrogen, partly linked to estrogen, or not linked to estrogen. In any event, clinicians rarely prescribe estrogen therapy for women who have a history of any type of breast cancer. Although the Women's Health Initiative study (see Question 81) of postmenopausal women indicates that there is a small increase in the risk of breast cancer when estrogen plus progestin is taken for more than 5 years, there is no evidence that taking HT causes a recurrence of breast cancer. In fact, both the American College of Obstetricians and the Society of Obstetricians and Gynaecologists of Canada say that women who were previously treated for breast cancer can consider ET or EPT use. Even so, few women opt for ET or EPT after breast cancer.

If your cancer was not estrogen-linked, and your hot flashes or sweats are very severe, your clinician may suggest you try a short course of hormone therapy. Or if your vaginal dryness is making you extremely uncomfortable, your clinician may prescribe a vaginal estrogen cream. This is really a quality-of-life decision that can only be made by you and your clinician together.

Some clinicians prescribe methyltestosterone (see Question 89 about androgens) for the treatment of moderate to severe hot flashes in women with a history of breast cancer, with the belief that testosterone will not increase the risk of breast cancer. But estrogenic effects are possible since testosterone is transformed into estrogen in the peripheral tissues, and in the Nurses Health Study, androgens did increase the risk of breast cancer to postmenopausal women.

Megace® (megaestrol acetate), a hormone treatment usually given to women with metastatic breast cancer, may be an option for you because it has also been found to relieve hot flashes. Ironically, Megace® is derived from progesterone. The use of **progestin therapy** alone for the treatment of hot flashes is not often used, but provides an option (see Question 77 about progestin-only therapy). The possible connection of progestin with breast cancer has been raised by the WHI research because combination estrogen and progestin increased the risk of breast cancer after 5 years, but estrogen alone did not.

Progestin therapy
progestin taken by itself for the treatment of menopausal symptoms.

The most widely used nonhormonal prescription treatment for hot flashes is antidepressants. Antidepressants are not currently approved by the FDA for the treatment of hot flashes, but have been widely studied and show beneficial effects on reducing hot flashes in women who were previously treated for breast cancer. See Questions 87 and 88 for nonhormone prescription treatments of hot flashes.

Some clinicians will discourage patients with breast cancer from taking soy supplements or phytoestrogens because of their unknown long-term effects on breast tissue. However, women who live in societies with high soy intake not only have fewer hot flashes, but are also less likely to develop breast cancer. While some clinicians will restrict soy intake in their patients with breast cancer, others say that women who already have breast cancer do not need to worry about eating soy in moderation.

Black cohosh has not been effective for the treatment of hot flashes in women with breast cancer who are also taking **tamoxifen**, a treatment often given to patients with breast cancer to prevent recurrence. Vitamin E is often recommended for treatment of hot flashes in women with a history of breast cancer. See the other questions and answers in Part 4, which will help you with alternative therapies and lifestyle management of your hot flashes.

For your vaginal symptoms, using a water-based vaginal lubricant or moisturizer or Vitamin E oil may help (see Question 66 about vaginal dryness). Because the exact amount of estrogen absorbed into the system from vaginal creams, the vaginal ring, or a vaginal suppository is not known, their use is still controversial among clinicians. Some vaginal options, like Vagifem® suppositories or Estring® ring, have lower amounts of hormones than others, and even very small amounts of estrogen can provide relief from the discomfort of vaginal dryness.

If you are having sexual problems in postmenopause, they are not likely a result of breast cancer. Breast cancer does not make you any more likely to have sexual problems than other women of the same age who do not have breast cancer.

Difficulty with memory and thinking can be particularly bothersome for women after treatment for breast cancer.

Tamoxifen

a medication often given to patients with estrogen-linked breast cancer to help prevent recurrence.

While memory changes can be related to stress or sleep changes from hot flashes and sweats, it can also be related to leftover nervous system effects from chemotherapy, and should be discussed with your clinician.

Prevention of osteoporosis is important for all women whether they have breast cancer or not. Calcium and magnesium taken together has shown some promise in relieving hot flashes, yet another option for controlling hot flashes in women with breast cancer. Evista® (raloxifene), used to prevent and treat bone loss, may also decrease the risk of estrogen-receptor positive breast cancer. However, Evista® may cause hot flashes. If you are already taking tamoxifen for breast cancer, you may get hot flashes and vaginal dryness but you are likely to also benefit from its bone protection.

Because weight gain during menopause and obesity have been associated with an increased risk of breast cancer, it is important to maintain a healthy weight to lower your risk of recurrence.

Sarah's comment:

OK—I'm in my late 40s and menopause starts—interrupted sleep, mood swings, irritability, and lack of concentration. After a couple years of it escalating, my doctor does a blood test and then puts me on Prempro! All of a sudden I'm human again—good sleep, smiling a lot, less tears—I should have been a poster child for this drug!!

Then WHAM—my yearly mammogram showed a mass. Followed by core biopsy, lumpectomy, and then 4 doses of chemotherapy and 42 radiation treatments. On top of the emotional trauma of being diagnosed with cancer, losing all my hair—"Q" ball, the lack of energy from the chemo/radiation and working full time—I wasn't allowed to go back on HRT or any natural estrogen. It felt like a death sentence!

Hot flashes, night sweats, skin changes—"liver spots" on my face, why couldn't they stay on my hands? Hair texture changes, lack of vaginal lubrication—they all came at me like an 18-wheeler. I remember when I was young, people would say that late middle-age women were "bitchy"—well, no wonder—who can keep a smile on her face and be pleasant when you're living on 2 or 3 hours of sleep a night and sleeping next to a man who falls asleep before his head hits the pillow and doesn't wake up until the alarm goes off!

I was determined to get all these negative life changes reversed and under control. First I tried various over-the-counter sleeping aids, and then had my doctor prescribe Trazodone that finally gave me 4-6 hours straight sleep plus being able to go back to sleep once I'd woken up with a hot flash. Began to feel normal—well, as normal as possible with "chemo brain"—but it took another couple years to "clear out all the cobwebs."

Not being able to take estrogen is still a negative—weight gain in all the wrong places, hair texture changes, the "spots," still having hot flashes but less often and less severe, lack of lubrication and sexual desire, etc.

Yes, slowly menopause is passing—regular sleep most of the time, less mood swings, more confident in myself, 5-years of a clean bill of health in regards to breast cancer. Now I can be a "red hat" lady with a smile on my face!

PART FIVE

Hormone Therapy and Other Treatment Options

What is hormone therapy? What are the benefits of HT? Why would I want to take it?

What questions should I ask my clinician when I am considering going on hormone therapy?

How can I manage the side effects from HT so that I don't have to stop taking it?

What other prescription medications might be effective for my symptoms?

More...

73. What is hormone therapy (HT)? What is estrogen therapy (ET)? What is progestin therapy (PT)? What is estrogen and progestin therapy (EPT)?

HT (hormone therapy) is an umbrella term that describes the use of estrogen, progesterone, or some combination of the two, and sometimes testosterone, to treat the symptoms of menopause. Technically, HT can also refer to other hormones for the treatment of cancer or other illnesses. For the purposes of this book, HT refers to the hormones used for managing menopausal symptoms in perimenopausal and postmenopausal women.

When estrogen is taken by itself without progestin, it is called estrogen therapy, or ET. When progestin is taken by itself without estrogen, it is called progestin therapy or PT. When estrogen and progestin are taken together, it is called estrogen-progestin therapy or EPT. ET, PT, and EPT are all forms of HT.

Estrogen taken daily causes the lining of the uterus (the endometrium) to thicken. Normally a menstrual period occurs when the built-up lining sheds. Adding progestin to estrogen to form a combination of hormones prevents the uterine lining from building up if taken every day, or causes it to come off and flow out just like a menstrual period if taken for 12 to 15 days of the cycle and then stopped. If the buildup of the lining is not prevented by progestin, overgrowth or endometrial hyperplasia can occur, which can lead to endometrial cancer. For this reason, ET alone is not prescribed for women who have their uterus. Instead EPT or PT is used to prevent overgrowth in the first place.

Estrogen therapy (ET) is available as pill, patch, cream, suppository, or gel. ET is usually taken daily to control menopausal symptoms and has several other beneficial effects (see Question 75 about benefits from HT).

There is no one right estrogen for every woman. Each woman has different cycles, different symptoms, different preferences about having a period or not, and different reactions to certain formulations. There are many types and formulations of both estrogen and progesterone, and sometimes your clinician will need to prescribe different types of estrogens and/or progesterones in different doses and combinations before you'll find the one that controls your symptoms with the fewest side effects.

- *Bio-identical estrogen* is made by taking steroid molecules from wild yam (an herb) or soy. "Bio-identical" means that the chemical structure of the manufactured estrogen is identical to estrogen produced naturally in your body, but bio-identical hormones are made in laboratories. These hormones are natural, like other forms of estrogen, since they are all made from plant or animal sources. Substances found in wild yam and soy are converted into the three types of estrogen made by the body (see Question 3 about estrogen). Estradiol (E2), in the form of **17-beta estradiol**, is the most commonly used bio-identical estrogen. The others are sometimes present in preparations, but as weaker estrogens they have less effect on symptoms than 17-beta estradiol. The three different types of estrogen can be prescribed in varying percentages by your clinician for compounding at a compounding

17-beta estradiol

the most commonly used bio-identical manufactured estrogen.

pharmacy. (e.g., Bi-Est, Tri-Est). Or, 17-beta estradiol can be prescribed alone (e.g., Estrace®), and is available at most regular pharmacies.

- *Conjugated equine estrogens (CEE)* are made using the estrogens found in the urine of pregnant mares. Although CEE is not bio-identical to your body's estrogens, it is a natural estrogen because it is made from an animal source, and like bio-identical estrogens, is made in a laboratory. CEE is one of the most prescribed and widely studied estrogens. It is absorbed well and is very effective for menopause symptom relief. CEE is found in such products as Premarin®, Prempro®, and Premphase®.

- *Synthetic conjugated estrogen* is made from plant sources and manufactured in the laboratory (e.g., Cenestin®).

- *Esterified estrogens* (Estratab® and Menest®), *estropipates* (Ogen®, Otho-Est®), and *ethinyl estradiol* (Estinyl®) are all synthesized estrogens. These estrogens are made by different processes, and may vary in how they are absorbed and in side effects that women experience.

Progestin therapy (PT), for the purposes of this book, refers to any progesterone that is manufactured and not made by the body. In pre-menopausal women, progestin is often given when periods are missed but there is no pregnancy (amenorrhea), to cause the uterine lining to shed like in a menstrual period. Progestin is also given to women who are taking estrogen to prevent a buildup of the uterine lining. Depending on the dose and how the progestin is taken (pills, IUD, gel, or cream), you might get a menstrual period, or what is more accurately called a "withdrawal bleed," because it happens after you stop taking, or withdraw, the prog-

Conjugated equine estrogen (CEE)

the most common form of estrogen used in hormone therapy (HT), a blend of estrogens extracted from the urine of pregnant mares.

Conjugated estrogen

a blend of several manufactured estrogens in one product used in HT.

Esterified estrogens estropipates, Ethinyl estradiol

a manufactured form of estrogen used in hormone therapy (HT).

estin. The progestin-containing IUD (Mirena®) is marketed and FDA-approved for birth control, but has also been used as a way to deliver progestin directly to the uterus in women who are taking estrogen-only preparations for their menopausal symptoms. Oral progestins can be taken daily or intermittently. Intermittent oral progestin will cause the uterine lining to shed like a period. Even though some studies show that progestin-only therapy can provide relief from hot flashes, PT is not usually the first choice for treating hot flashes. See Question 77 about using progesterone to treat hot flashes.

Some forms of progestin can be purchased without a prescription, but most need to be prescribed by your clinician. Unlike estrogen, there are no animal sources of progestins. The following forms of progestins are made by taking steroid molecules from plants like wild yam and soy.

- *Bio-identical progesterone* is sometimes called "natural" progesterone, although technically all progestins are natural because they are made from plants. Bio-identical progesterone comes in powder form called **micronized** *progesterone* (e.g., Prometrium®), and is available in pill or vaginal suppository form. The suppositories are compounded and are usually used for pregnant women when extra progesterone is needed for a healthy pregnancy. The pills are available at both compounding pharmacies and regular pharmacies, but insurance companies may not pay for prescriptions at compounding pharmacies. If you are allergic to peanuts, you should never take Prometrium® capsules because they have peanut oil in them. Prometrium® can cause dizziness at first,

Micronized

when a product is prepared with very small particle sizes, as opposed to fewer larger particles, so it has a larger surface area and is better absorbed in the intestines.

so it is a good idea to take it at bedtime. Some clinicians prescribe Prometrium® to be taken twice a day; others prescribe it for once a day. Prometrium® may have fewer side effects for some women and may not increase cholesterol levels like other progestins can. Bio-identical progesterone can also be made into creams at compounding pharmacies.

- Some "progesterone" creams are available without a prescription. These products have varying amounts of progestin in them and are not regulated by the FDA like prescription products are. The amount of progesterone actually absorbed from progesterone cream can vary from woman to woman. Some nonprescription wild yam creams state they contain progesterone. Some do and some don't. Your body cannot convert wild yam into progesterone—that has to be done in a laboratory.

- Other *synthetic progestins* include *medroyxyprogesterone acetate* (Provera®, Cycrin®), *norethindrone acetate* (Aygestin®, Femhrt®, Activella®), *norethindrone* (Micronor®, NorQD®), and *norgestimate* (Ortho-Prefest®). These progestins are made in a laboratory and are chemically different from each other, and the side effects experienced by an individual woman might be different as well. Sometimes, you will need to try several progestins before you find the one that is best for you.

Because progestins are used to prevent overgrowth of the uterine lining, some women who are taking estrogen alone have used a nonprescription progesterone cream, thinking it will provide that protection. But progesterone creams, even prescription creams, do not provide high enough blood levels of progesterone to offer any protection. You need to take a progestin by mouth, use a combination patch (with both estrogen and progestin), or use the Mirena® IUD.

Estrogen-progestin therapy (EPT) is a combination of estrogen and progestin used for menopause symptoms in women who have a uterus. EPT can be created by combining ET and PT products, and is available in several forms including pill, patch, cream, gel, vaginal ring, and IUD. Estrogen and progestin given together tend to give slightly better relief from hot flashes than estrogen alone, so lower doses of each can be used. There are many different schedules for taking EPT, some have a scheduled period (withdrawal bleed) every month or every few months, and others have minimal or no menstrual bleeding. The decision about what is best for you is based on many things, like your preference for having a period or not, and other medical conditions that you might have. You should discuss all of the options with your clinician and make a decision together about which is best for you. See Appendix B for a list of various hormone therapy products.

74. Why was HRT (hormone replacement therapy) changed to HT (hormone therapy)?

HRT (hormone replacement therapy) was the name initially given to combined estrogen and progestin treatment because it was believed that estrogen and progestin needed to be "replaced" after menopause. The earlier thinking was that if the body was losing estrogen and progestin at menopause, then they should be replaced so that the body would remain in its "natural" state. It was also thought that the estrogen and progestin that was replaced would match up with the estrogen and progesterone receptors so that menopausal symptoms would stop.

It was also believed that some of the negative health effects that happen after menopause could be reversed by replacing the "lost" estrogen and progesterone. Since the loss of estrogen is associated with increased risks of heart disease, bone loss, skin changes, memory changes, changes in metabolism, emotional changes, and a lower sense of well-being, many thought that "replacing" lost estrogen would prevent or reverse these processes.

During the summer of 2002, the FDA changed the terms used to more accurately reflect the concept of hormone therapies. Using "replacement" as part of HRT suggested that menopause was creating a deficiency of something that had to be replaced. This was contrary to the notion that menopause is a normal life event. While the symptoms of menopause can be bothersome and uncomfortable, menopause remains a natural process. So, the FDA decided to change HRT to the more accurate term hormone therapy (HT). The change reflects the idea that hormones can be given to increase a woman's well-being, rather than replace hormones in which she is deficient.

75. What are the benefits of HT? Why would I want to take it?

You would take it to control your menopause related symptoms and feel better. If you are having moderate to severe symptoms that are wreaking havoc with your quality of life, then HT might be an appropriate choice for you. The major benefit to HT is that it is the single most effective way to relieve the many symptoms of menopause, especially hot flashes. Sleep is improved as a direct result of HT, with fewer hot flashes or night sweats that wake you. Women who take HT fall asleep faster, have more time in deep sleep, and wake less often during the night. Getting more sleep means you feel less irritable, you cope better with stress when you are awake, and your ability to focus, concentrate, and remember is better.

Women report real benefits to their concentration, memory, and thinking processes while taking HT. They feel more connected, they remember things better, and they can concentrate better. Some of these benefits may be due to sleeping better, but they could be a result of the HT itself. Estrogen's beneficial effect on mental function is linked to receptors in the **hippocampus**, the part of the brain that helps with memory. Estrogen seems to be helpful if you take it right when you enter menopause, but taking it several years after menopause could make dementia worse. This is also true of heart disease. Many studies show some protection against heart disease when HT is taken at the time of menopause; i.e., estrogens reduce the "bad" cholesterol (LDL) and increase the "good" cholesterol (HDL). Recent studies showed, however, an increase in heart disease when it was taken by older women.

Hippocampus
a part of the brain that helps with memory.

Some forms of HT also help with urinary incontinence and vaginal dryness, and can improve sexual function. Vaginal dryness is relieved by HT, so sex is better. All women experience vaginal dryness as they age, but the severity is individual. It can range from "no big deal," to "it hurts to sit," or anywhere in between. HT used either throughout the system (patch, pills, or gel) or in the vagina (cream, suppository, or ring) will replenish the skin cells inside the vagina that die off during postmenopause. After you take estrogen for a while, you will have better lubrication and response during sex. HT also improves sexual satisfaction, and not only because you are more comfortable—you might also be more interested in sex and might have better orgasms. Urinary leakage and infection can get better, too, because HT helps tone the muscles that control urination.

Estrogen also helps retain tone in your skin and reduce the appearance of wrinkles by increasing the amount of collagen, or supportive tissue, under the skin surface. It increases the thickness and improves the elasticity of your skin, and helps to retain skin moisture, further improving its appearance. And, women who use HT are less likely to develop that "apple" shape, since they don't get as much extra fat around their middles. So, if you are feeling wrinkled and old on top of your sleepless nights and hot flashes, taking estrogen might help you feel better about how you look.

HT can also help your appearance by preventing bone loss and the hunched appearance that goes along with bone loss in the spine (see Question 39 about bone loss). You will be less likely to break a bone if you take ET or EPT, not only because it helps to strengthen bones, but because it helps you keep your balance so you are less likely to fall in the first place. ET and EPT also helps to prevent tooth loss and inflammation of the gums. Even though ET and EPT have great protective effects against bone loss, they usually aren't used solely for that reason. If you are lucky enough not to have moderate to severe symptoms, then other treatment options for protecting your bones might be better (see Table 7).

There are other benefits from taking HT as well. EPT may lower your risk of colon cancer, but taking estrogen alone may not. Estrogen may also help preserve vision as you age.

The reasons most women take HT are to treat hot flashes and to improve their sense of well-being and quality of life. Research studies confirm that women with moderate to severe symptoms have a better quality of life when taking HT. When hot flashes continue well into your postmenopause years, HT's benefits probably start to look better. But you don't really need research to convince you. You will know if you feel better!

Karin's comment:

Hormones changed my life. I couldn't sleep, couldn't think, never had sex—I was so depressed! I was afraid of trying hormones but nothing else was working. I tried the vitamins and the cohosh stuff, but it didn't make a difference. So I finally talked to my clinician about it. She said I didn't need to suffer and she encouraged me to try hormones. So I did. And I am so glad! I am back to my old self. I feel good and am on top of things at work, and my husband is glad too—he told me that I wasn't the same woman he had fallen in love with, and he is so glad that I am back! I am not going to go off them—I don't ever want to go back to being such a mess.

Emily's comment:

After almost a year with no periods the hot flashes and night sweats were becoming unbearable. There was never

*an undisrupted night. I had had some improvement with
1000 mg of calcium, then 1500 mg per day initially, but
that relief was in the past; likewise with Estroven and
Remifemin. I was the perfect candidate for HT, even with
a family history of breast cancer. I exercise three times a
week, walk daily, have a great HDL/total cholesterol ratio,
and had recently lost ten pounds. My provider started me
on 0.5 mg of estradiol and it was like a switch had gone off
(or on). The night sweats stopped almost completely, the
flashes were back to a manageable level, but most amazing
of all, my cognition improved dramatically. The changes
had been subtle, so I did not even know it had been off.
Also, I would never have described myself as having been
depressed. But after beginning the estrogen I was able to
generate several articles in just days—this after staring at
the computer for weeks without writing much. Progestin
will be added to the mix in a week, to protect the lining of
my uterus, and then we will re-evaluate my doses. I have
always been an advocate of HT, especially for hot
flashes/sweats; however, the personal benefits that I have
realized have increased my advocacy even more. Thank
goodness for all of the options we now have available.*

76. How does HT work? Is HT only available in tablet form?

Hormones are processed in the liver. The estrogen that
you take in pill form is processed so it can get into your
bloodstream and bind with the receptors all over your
body. When this happens, your body will think it has
more estrogen, and your menopausal symptoms such as
hot flashes, night sweats, or vaginal dryness will either
go away or at least decrease. It takes about a week for
your blood level of hormones to balance out after you
start taking it. But it can take up to 6 weeks to see a

full difference in symptoms because it takes a while for the estrogen to match up with enough receptor sites.

Hormones can also be taken by applying them to your skin in patches, creams, gel, or by vaginal rings or suppositories. The patches, pills, gel, body creams, and one type of vaginal ring (Femring®) provide hormones that are absorbed into the bloodstream in high enough amounts to have effects all over the body. The vaginal creams, suppositories (Vagifem®), and other vaginal rings (Estring®) provide hormones mostly at the vagina; little is absorbed into the system.

Patches are available with estrogen alone, or in a combination of estrogen and progestin. Patches are usually applied once or twice a week to a different spot on your lower abdomen, thigh, or buttocks. The biggest drawback to using a patch is the adhesive, which is similar to the adhesive used in Band-Aids®, and can be irritating to the skin. Estrogen is also available in creams or gel, and progestin is available in creams. Estrogen and progestin creams that are put into the vagina can be messy and leak out when you stand up, so using them at bedtime is best. The applicators used to put in creams or suppositories can hurt when you first use them, but it gets better with time as the estrogen is absorbed and the tissue is not as dry. Also, you can insert the suppository using your finger, rather than the applicator.

Estrogen gel is rubbed into the skin on your arm just like a lotion. Estrogen cream is rubbed into your thigh the same way. To avoid irritation where you apply patches, gel, or cream, and to make sure they are absorbed well, you should wash and dry the area before you apply it. You should not use other creams, lotions, or perfumes in the area.

Vaginal rings are made of clear plastic and are worn in the vagina much like a diaphragm. They have different doses of estrogen in them that is slowly released over 3 months. At the end of 3 months, you remove it and put in a new one. You can leave your ring in during sex; your partner usually can't feel it. The biggest drawback to using a ring is that you need to feel comfortable about putting it in and removing it from the vagina yourself. The vaginal rings can be uncomfortable for the first few days, but usually are not even felt. You don't need to measure out a dose if you use a ring because a standard amount of estrogen is released over time. The ring can also be helpful if you have stress incontinence because it gives gentle support in the vagina.

When hormones are absorbed through the skin (topically), they are not processed by the liver in the same way that oral hormones are. Instead, the hormones are absorbed right into the bloodstream through the skin, so you can take a lower dose. Since you have receptors all over your body, hormones have many effects besides helping with your menopause symptoms. For example, hormones can change levels of cholesterol and triglycerides and affect how your body uses insulin. Estrogen also increases your risk for developing a blood clot. By taking a hormone that is absorbed through the skin, some of these other effects are reduced or altered, so it can be a better choice if you have high blood pressure, diabetes, or take medicines that affect the liver.

Vaginal creams, suppositories, and the rings are extremely helpful for urinary and genital symptoms.

Vaginal creams can be used intermittently, and the amount of cream that you use can be adjusted to your symptoms. You may find that you need to use a lot less cream over time to still get good relief from dryness. You can also take oral estrogen pills for vaginal symptoms, but the reverse isn't usually true. Vaginal creams and suppositories give excellent relief of vaginal symptoms, but do not usually provide enough estrogen to prevent hot flashes. The amount of estrogen released in your blood from vaginal creams or suppositories is extremely small compared to oral estrogen, or estrogen patches or gel. When full doses of vaginal estrogen creams or suppositories are used, some women may get hot flash relief and some prevention for bone loss, but that isn't common. When the full dose is used in women who have their uterus, a progestin is usually still needed. It's not clear whether progestin is needed when less cream or fewer suppositories are used. Vaginal creams can be applied using an applicator, or just placed onto your finger and rubbed gently onto the vagina walls.

Some women with very severe symptoms might need to take estrogen pills, patch, body cream, or gel along with vaginal cream at first. Vaginal cream and suppositories can give you immediate relief for vaginal dryness, and the patch, pill, or gel will help with hot flashes over time. The vaginal cream or suppositories can be stopped once the patch, pill, body cream, or gel takes effect, usually by about 6 weeks.

ET alone is usually started as one pill per day, one patch every few days, or gel or cream applied every day. ET alone is only prescribed for women without a uterus. Some women will take their estrogen pill every day, and others will only need it every other day. If you skip your estrogen for a couple of days and your symptoms return, you'll know that you need to take it more often. But if you miss two doses and don't have a lot of bothersome symptoms, then you may be able to take it or use it less often. This applies to estrogen and oral EPT. If you have been taking combination daily EPT for long enough, you are not likely to get bleeding if you take it every other day. You need to discuss with your clinician any changes you are considering in how you take your HT.

If you have a uterus and you are taking hormones, it's important to take progestin as part of your regimen. Progestin will keep the buildup of the uterine lining to a very minimal amount if you take it daily, every other day, or in a pulsed fashion (3 days of ET, then 3 days of EPT in a repeated pattern, e.g., Prefest®). Or, progestin will cause the built-up lining to shed so you get a period after you take it for 12 to 15 days. Some women, after taking HT for several years, will not get periods, even after taking progestin. If this happens, you should discuss it with your clinician. You will still need to take the progestin to prevent buildup of the lining, but you may be able to take it less often.

There are four types of oral regimens for EPT:

The **cyclic regimen** is one in which a woman takes an estrogen tablet once a day for 25 days of the month. For the last 10 to 14 days of estrogen, she adds a progestin tablet, and takes both estrogen and progestin pills each day until day 25 of the month. This regimen mimics the way your body makes estrogen and progesterone, and is similar to how hormones are taken in many birth control pills. Since you have stopped your

Cyclic regimen

a method of taking hormone therapy (HT) in which the woman takes an estrogen tablet once a day for 25 days of the month. For the last 10 to 14 days of estrogen, she adds a progestin tablet, and takes both estrogen and progestin pills each day until day 25 of the month. She takes nothing from day 26 to the end of the month.

menstrual periods, the calendar month is used to start the estrogen on the first day of the month. This regimen is not common because the symptoms you are trying to relieve usually come back when you are not taking any hormones, meaning day 26 to day 30 or 31 of the calendar month. If you try the cyclic regimen and don't get a relapse of your symptoms during the days you are off the estrogen, then you probably don't need to be on EPT to control your symptoms.

In the **sequential cyclic regimen**, a woman takes estrogen every day, and adds a progestin on days 1 through 14 or days 14 through 28. Once the progestin is stopped, she gets a period. Some women don't like the side effects of progestin, which may include bloating, moodiness, headaches, and breast tenderness. Sometimes progestin is only prescribed every few months, causing a period only four times a year. It is unclear at this time how often a woman needs to have a period to prevent overgrowth of the uterine lining. The recommendation is that you have a "regular" withdrawal bleed, but whether the bleed is once a month or once every few months is up to you and your clinician. Premphase® is an example of sequential cyclic EPT. Sequential cyclic EPT can also be prescribed by combining estrogen (e.g., Premarin®, 17-beta estradiol) and progestin (e.g., Provera®, Prometrium®) products.

The **continuous combined regimen** was developed for women who don't want to have periods. In this case, estrogen and progestin are taken every day without a break. The progestin, when taken daily with the estrogen, prevents the endometrial lining from building up, so regular periods are not needed. Some women don't like the continuous combined regimen because of the side effects from progestin. Femhrt®,

Sequential cyclic regimen

a method of taking hormone therapy (HT) in which the woman takes estrogen every day continuously, and adds a progestin on days 1 through 14 or days 14 through 28. She has a period after she finishes taking the progestin every month.

Continuous combined regimen

a method of taking hormone therapy (HT) in which the woman takes estrogen and progestin every day without stopping.

Activella®, and Prempro® are examples of this regimen. Continuous combined EPT can also be prescribed by combining estrogen and progestin products.

Pulsed regimen

a method of taking hormone therapy (HT) in which estrogen is taken for 3 days, and then progestin is added to the estrogen for 3 days, then estrogen alone for 3 days, and then estrogen with progestin for 3 days, and so on, in a repeated fashion.

The **pulsed regimen** was developed as an alternative to the continuous combined. In this regimen, estrogen is taken for 3 days, and then progestin is added to the estrogen for 3 days, then estrogen alone for 3 days, and then estrogen with progestin for 3 days, and so on. Prefest® is an example of a pulsed regimen. If you choose this regimen, you might get more breakthrough bleeding.

Even if you select a regimen that is designed to avoid withdrawal bleeds, it is very likely that you will experience breakthrough bleeding during the first few months. In fact, the single most common side effect from taking EPT is breakthrough bleeding, especially in the first 3 to 4 months. Many women will experience breakthrough bleeding throughout the first year of EPT. Some women mistakenly believe that if they are still getting a period on HT, they are fertile. This is not true: HT does not make you ovulate, so you cannot get pregnant. HT only provides enough hormones to reduce your symptoms and prevent buildup of the uterine lining. However, if you are placed on HT before you have gone 1 year without periods, you may ovulate and can get pregnant. If this is the case, you must use an alternate method of birth control because the dose of the hormones in HT is not high enough to prevent pregnancy. Taking a birth control pill is often a good option for women who are perimenopausal, and who want hormones for symptom management. If you cannot get pregnant (e.g., you had your tubes tied or your partner had a vasectomy), then HT is an appropriate option to consider.

The dose of the hormones in HT is not high enough to prevent pregnancy.

Remember that you can respond differently to different types of estrogens and progestins, so let your clinician know if you are having bothersome side effects. A change in your prescription might be needed. See Table 14 for managing side effects of hormone therapy.

Some women can't tolerate the side effects of progestin. Another option is to take estrogen by pill, patch, body cream, or gel, and use an IUD that has progestin (Mirena®) in it. The progestin in the IUD has an effect in the uterus to prevent overgrowth, but isn't absorbed into the bloodstream enough to cause annoying side effects like bloating, tender breasts, and mood changes. Irregular bleeding rarely continues after a few months because the progestin in the IUD prevents the uterine lining from building up much. The Mirena® IUD is put into the uterus by your clinician and may stay in for up to 5 years. If you don't need to keep taking estrogen for symptoms, the IUD can also be removed. This IUD is an excellent choice for birth control during perimenopause because it can be combined with a lower dose of estrogen to control symptoms like hot flashes and night sweats. This way, birth control pills that have higher doses of estrogen are not needed.

77. I understand that progesterone alone has been used to treat hot flashes. Is that true?

Yes. Progestin therapies are getting more attention as an option for women who can't or won't use estrogen. Several research studies show that progestin injections (depot-medroxyprogesterone, Depo-Provera®) or pills (medroxyprogesterone acetate, MPA and megestrol acetate, Megace®) can help with hot flashes without using estrogen.

Progesterone is also available in creams such as Phytogest®, Endocreme®, Meno Cream®, Pro-Gest®, and Pro-Dermex®. Although some studies of progesterone creams showed a decrease in hot flashes, others showed no change. Progesterone creams do not protect you from bone loss, and do not provide high enough blood levels of progesterone hormone to protect the uterine lining from overgrowth if you are taking estrogen.

The amount of progesterone in the creams varies from 2 to 700 mg per ounce, and how much you will absorb through your skin can vary as well. These creams are regulated as dietary supplements, so they are not held to the same standards as prescription medications. The manufacturing processes and contents in individual creams can vary.

Progesterone creams and gels can also be prescribed through a compounding pharmacy. Some of these creams have the same names as the nonprescription varieties, but are held to the FDA standards for prescription medicines. Progesterone creams or gels are massaged into the skin at the breasts, upper arms, or thighs, and usual doses are ½ to 1 teaspoon once or twice a day, and a break for a week once a month may be recommended. Progesterone, when taken in pill form, can cause unpleasant side effects like bloating, nausea, headache, and breast tenderness, but absorption through the skin can reduce many of these.

More study is needed to determine if progestin therapies will prove to be a safe and effective option. It certainly can't hurt to discuss progestin therapies with your clinician while you're considering all of the options for managing your symptoms.

78. What are the side effects of HT? Are there circumstances when HT is not an option? Given all the controversy about HT, is it safe to take for my symptoms? I am having a terrible time with hot flashes, night sweats, poor sleep, and vaginal dryness, which makes me very uncomfortable all the time. Should I ignore the risks of HT and improve the quality of my life?

Most package inserts with prescription medications contain a long list of complications, risks, side effects, and adverse events. Luckily, few people actually experience serious side effects, but they are listed so you know what to watch for, just in case. There are risks and possible side effects for every medication, herb, vitamin, or dietary supplement you take or apply to your skin. The risks and side effects listed here are intended to give you enough information to make an informed decision (with advice from your clinician) about using estrogen and progesterone for your menopause symptoms. Because of all the research that has been done on estrogen and progestins, we know much more about potential risks and benefits for these therapies than we do for many other medications and supplements.

There are risks and possible side effects for every medication, herb, vitamin, or dietary supplement you take or apply to your skin.

Common side effects from estrogen can include vaginal bleeding or spotting, slight breast enlargement or thickening, breast soreness, bloating or cramps, weight changes, nausea, and vomiting. Other effects might include headache, swelling, high blood pressure, hair thinning or increased hair growth, rash, vaginal yeast infections, vision changes, or difficulty wearing contact lenses. See Question 83 about managing the side effects of hormone therapy. The increased breast tissue density might make it harder for a radiologist to read your mammogram, but this effect goes away if you come off HT. Changes in cholesterol are common, too, but most of these are good—estrogen decreases total cholesterol and the "bad" cholesterol (LDL), and increases the "good" cholesterol (HDL). Because estrogen can interfere with insulin use in the body, it can also increase blood sugar levels and triglyceride levels. But combined estrogen and progestin may reduce the likelihood of developing diabetes. Other side effects include return of cervical mucous secretion, improved mood or mood changes, and changes in libido—these can be good things!

The possible risks and serious reactions to estrogen are uncommon, and include things like depression, uterine fibroid growth, worsening of asthma, blood clots, stroke, heart attack, dementia, cancers of the breast, ovary, or uterine lining, or problems with the gallbladder, liver, or pancreas. The risk of breast cancer increases after you have been on estrogen-progestin therapy for over 5 years, but the risk does not stay with you once you have stopped taking it.

Serious risks to taking progestins are also rare and include blood clots, stroke, heart attack, breast cancer, high blood pressure, or problems with the liver or gallbladder.

Common side effects from progestins can include nausea, breast tenderness, fluid retention, weight changes, headache, or depressed mood. Other side effects might include rash, itching, increased body hair, hair loss, appetite changes, or acne. In higher doses it can cause the breasts to produce milk (**lactation**), as it does naturally following pregnancy. Progestins can cause missed periods (this is the goal when you take the continuous combined regimen of estrogen-progestin therapy) and may also affect your sex drive.

Lactation

the period of time when the mammary glands in the breasts produce milk.

You must never take estrogen or progestin if you are allergic to it. Do not take Prometrium® capsules if you are allergic to peanuts, as they contain peanut oil. Estrogen or progestin are also not generally recommended if you have vaginal or uterine bleeding that has not been checked by your clinician, breast cancer, any estrogen-linked cancer, blood clots or history of blood clots in the veins, blood clots in the arteries in the past 12 months, pregnancy, or liver problems.

Under some circumstances, your clinician may still recommend estrogen or estrogen-progestin therapy for you even if you have a contraindication such as breast cancer. Sometimes symptoms can be too severe without hormone therapy. Sometimes the quality of life trumps warning labels. But you must engage in an active discussion, ask questions, get answers, and make an informed decision with your clinician before you take estrogen or progesterone.

Jackie's comment:

About 12 years ago, the doctor gave me some hormones, but after a month, I did not like how I was feeling. I was bloated and my breasts hurt all the time. We tried cutting the dosage in half and we tried the patch. I think I gained weight. I just didn't feel comfortable. After six months, I said I couldn't take it anymore and I stopped the hormones completely. Within a week, I felt normal again.

Paula's comment:

I am happy to see that I am not the only one who has decided after reading the actual statistics that I am going to take HRT (Estratest®) anyway—in my case even though I have DCIS [ductal carcinoma in-situ]. Both my grandmothers had breast cancer and radical mastectomies. They both lived to be very old ladies (94 and 85) and had never taken HT. I have had three lumpectomies since December 24, 2003 and now, after three surgeries, I still must have the breast removed. If I get it in the other one, I will wait until it progresses, if it does, to have any surgery. I understood too late that some in the medical profession do not even consider DCIS to be cancer.

Since my HRT was cut back drastically last summer, I have developed dry eye syndrome (had to see an ophthalmologist for treatment), have had 6 months of seborrheic dermatitis on my face, and still have rosacea, for which I am seeing a dermatologist weekly; have a very dry vagina (my gyn could not take a proper pap smear and had started me on an estrogen cream to clear up things, when the scare tactics finally became so great that he took me off that as well as anything by mouth). Sex has become almost impossible. It is very painful and I bleed afterwards. I really love my husband and would rather not get a divorce. I went to see my gynecologist and discussed this with him. I told him that one way or another I am going back on some amount of HT. Apparently a woman's overall health and well-

being does not occur to, or count with, some in the medical profession.

As it happens, my gynecologist (a very well known and highly thought of specialist) was very supportive, and we worked things out in a way that will let me live a relatively normal life. He must be in his late 60s and he even told me his own wife still takes estrogen. He also explained how the statistics have been distorted to make it look like the percentage of breast cancer in older women is going up, when actually the control group's numbers had taken a blip dive downward, which then made the percentage of difference look greater. In reality the older women's numbers had not really changed in any significant way. One is forced to wonder whose axes are being ground here.

79. What questions should I ask my clinician when I am considering going on hormone therapy?

The decision to use HT is an individual one. You must weigh the possible risks against the possible benefits. See Questions 75, 78, and 81 discussing risks, benefits, and controversy about HT. Each woman is different. What you can tolerate in terms of symptoms may not be what another woman could handle. What you're willing to risk may be different from what your best friend is willing to risk. And, what you and your best friend are at risk for is likely different, as well. Remember: Hormones are not miracle drugs. They may not instantly relieve your symptoms. You may relieve one symptom, yet get another one as a side effect of the hormones. But you might also have drier clothes and a good night's sleep.

You must weigh the possible risks against the possible benefits.

Try answering the following questions yourself before discussing HT with your clinician:

- What is the severity of my symptoms? How frequently do they occur? Do they interfere with my work or enjoyment of the activities of daily living?
- Have I kept track of things that bring on symptoms and tried to eliminate them (e.g., stopped eating chocolate if it brings on a hot flash)?
- What changes have I made in my lifestyle to reduce my symptoms? (See Table 13.)
- Am I trying to live in healthier ways (e.g., quit smoking)?
- What am I not willing or able to do at this time to modify my life? What is available to help for the short term and the long term?
- In addition to lifestyle changes, have I tried using vitamins and mineral supplements to help with my symptoms?
- Do I have any medical conditions that would make it unsafe for me to go on HT? Am I taking any medications that would interact badly with HT?
- If I go on hormones, what would be the best route of administration for me? Will I be able to develop a regimen of remembering to take pills? Will I be willing to change patches? Will I be willing to apply vaginal cream or insert a vaginal ring?
- Will I be comfortable knowing that there are risks to taking estrogen and progesterone? Do I understand that all medications, vitamins, herbs, and supplements carry certain risks?
- Do I understand the benefits of estrogen in addition to relieving menopausal symptoms, such as reducing the risk of bone loss and colon cancer?

- Do I understand the side effects of hormone therapy? Do I understand that one symptom may be relieved by the hormones and that I may get another symptom as a result of the hormones?
- If I took hormones and I stopped having severe hot flashes, how happy would I be? If the symptoms could be relieved by hormones, do I think my life would be much better?
- Do I understand that taking hormones does not mean that I will get breast cancer? And do I also understand that not taking hormones in no way prevents me from getting breast cancer?

If you are interested in HT, schedule an appointment to have a discussion about HT with your clinician. You should make sure the following questions are answered before you leave with your prescription:

- How long will I be on this?
- What symptoms should I report to you?
- When do you want to see me again?
- What are the options if I choose not to take this?
- How long will it be before I notice any improvement or change?
- What side effects or symptoms should I watch for? How can I minimize or prevent these?
- Will side effects or symptoms decrease with time?
- If I don't like taking it, should I let you know I have stopped it?
- What do I do if I miss a dose?
- What if I go out of town and forget my prescription at home? Will it be a problem if I miss a week? A month?
- Is there a specific time of day I should take my medications?

- Will HT interact with other medications that I'm taking?
- Are there other nonprescription medicines, herbs, or diet supplements that I should not take with HT?
- Can I still drink alcohol?

Madeline's comment:

At the time my symptoms started, my doctor asked me if I wanted estrogen. I told him that if I could do without it, that's what I'd prefer. Back in the early 1990s, there was also controversy about taking hormones. My mother took estrogen for a long time. I remember one of her hot flashes at Christmas before she went on estrogen. She went outside, stood in the snow bank, and lifted her long holiday skirt right up! I told myself that if my symptoms interfered with my life, then I would take the estrogen too. I felt that my symptoms were minimal. Occasionally my husband would disagree! I had hot flashes for 10 years before I was finally done with them.

80. Are there tests that need to be done before I take HT? How about while I'm taking it?

Yes. Whether you choose to use HT or not, you should have a complete history, physical exam with height and weight measures, and pelvic exam, as well as the routine screening tests recommended for your age (see Table 3 about screening recommendations for midlife women). These routine tests most likely include blood pressure screening, a mammogram, a cervical Pap test, and blood tests for thyroid function, cholesterol levels, and blood sugar after fasting. None of these tests are required before you start taking HT.

But it is a good idea to have all of your screening tests updated before you begin any new type of therapy. Screening tests for colon cancer and bone density may also be recommended depending on your age and risks. After you have been on HT for about 6 to 12 weeks, some clinicians will want to test for thyroid levels and blood sugar if you have a thyroid disorder or diabetes because HT can sometimes interact with medications used for these conditions. Most clinicians will also monitor cholesterol levels more closely while you are on HT.

Your clinician might check your "maturational index" to see how many surface cells are present in the vagina. This can be useful when your primary symptom is vaginal dryness or pain during intercourse. It can help your clinician distinguish between estrogen loss or other problems as the cause of your symptoms. If you don't have very many surface cells, estrogen cream applied to the vaginal tissue is most likely to help.

Estrogen or progesterone levels in the blood or saliva are rarely measured before you take HT or after you have been on it. Instead, your symptoms are monitored. If your symptoms get better and you feel good, then you are getting enough. If you miss a day or two and your symptoms don't come back, you might be able to use a lower dose. Most clinicians will review your symptoms and dose every year. Hormones, like all other medicine, should be taken in the lowest dose that works.

When you are taking testosterone, it is slightly different. Testosterone levels are often checked before and while you are taking testosterone.

81. There has been a lot of controversy about HT recently. Why is that? Why is the Women's Health Initiative so important to the evaluation of HT?

The controversy is about whether HT does more harm than good: Do the benefits of using HT outweigh the risks, or do the risks outweigh the benefits? This controversy has been developing over time, and became much more pronounced when part of the Women's Health Initiative (WHI) study was stopped 3 years earlier than planned in 2002 because the risks exceeded the benefits of estrogen-progestin therapy for the study participants.

The WHI is a 15-year study looking at whether hormone use (estrogen-progestin therapy [Prempro®] or estrogen therapy [Premarin®]) or diet (low fat or calcium plus vitamin D) reduces the risk for heart disease, breast cancer, colon cancer, and broken bones due to bone loss in postmenopausal women. WHI also monitored for strokes and blood clots. The study was started in 1991, and the part evaluating EPT was stopped in 2002 because the risks (having heart disease, stroke, blood clots, and invasive breast cancer) were calculated to be higher than the benefits (lower rates of colon cancer and fewer broken bones due to bone loss).

When the EPT part of the study was stopped early, there was heavy news coverage, and many women immediately stopped their hormones because they were afraid they would get heart disease, breast cancer, or have a stroke. Some of this was related to the way the statistics were reported in the news. Statistics are not easy to understand—the numbers can make it sound like the risks or benefits are much bigger than they actually are. For example, the media reported that there was a 26% increase in the risk of getting breast cancer and a 29% risk for heart disease while taking EPT. Even though these percentages sound high, the actual numbers show that the risk for an individual woman is very low. The 26% for breast cancer refers to the comparison between the number of women who would get breast cancer if they took hormones (38 out of 10,000) versus the number who would get breast cancer if they did not take hormones (30 out of 10,000). So, 8 more women out of 10,000 would get breast cancer; 38 is 26% higher than 30, hence the 26%. The individual risk is quite low (<1%). The same is true for heart disease: In groups of 10,000 women, 7 more would develop heart disease in a year on versus those off hormones. Again, the individual risk is very low (<1%).

In 2004, the estrogen-only part of the WHI study was stopped, about 1 year earlier than planned. It was stopped because the risk for stroke was higher in women using estrogen than in those who were not using it, and because the researchers did not think they would learn more by continuing the study for an additional year. In this part of the study, taking estrogen did not change the risk for heart disease, colon cancer, or breast cancer, but it did reduce the risk for breaking a hip.

Following the first news reports, there were many people who tried to analyze and understand the WHI results. Over time, three "camps" have formed in the controversy: those who think the results are faulty, those who think HT is too risky for any woman to take, and those who are in the middle. Some in the first camp have commented about the way that the study was designed, suggesting that since the participants did not have notable menopause symptoms, and were on average 63 years of age, the results don't apply to younger women who are entering menopause and having moderate to severe symptoms. They reason that benefits cannot be measured in the WHI study because the main reason for using HT was not evaluated (women with notable symptoms were excluded from the WHI study because they would have known they were receiving hormones and not a placebo when their symptoms stopped). Some wonder if the findings in the WHI study apply to other types of estrogens and progestins. But the FDA required *all* prescription estrogen and estrogen-progestin products, not just those used in the study, to change their labels to reflect the risks identified in the WHI. The risk for breast cancer has also been questioned since it did not increase in the estrogen-only part of the WHI. Another controversy that arose from the estrogen-progestin therapy results centers on the length of time that breast cancer takes to develop. It generally takes 7 to 8 years to develop breast cancer; how then could estrogen-progestin therapy taken for 5 years be responsible for the increase in breast cancer?

Those in the second camp say that the evidence showing that risks are greater than benefits is too strong to ignore—women should not use HT. Still others in the third camp think that the WHI did show important information about hormone use. They say the WHI results do need to be considered with women who are interested in using hormones for their symptoms— decisions about using hormones or not must be made individually based on a woman's risks, symptoms, and life situation.

As a result of the WHI studies, some clinicians advised their patients to stop both EPT and ET. Others were more reluctant to take patients off the best-known treatment for moderate to severe **vasomotor** symptoms of menopause. Still others decided to continue to recommend that their patients be on HT for no more than 5 years. The response by women was similar. Some stopped immediately and found their symptoms were minimal. Others found they did not feel well off the medications and resumed them. It should be stressed that none of the approaches are incorrect, but they all should be discussed with your clinician.

On one thing, everyone agrees: Recommendations about using hormones have changed. In the mid-1990s, the U.S. Preventive Services Task Force, a government group charged with evaluating scientific studies to determine screening, diagnostic, and treatment recommendations, recommended that all postmenopausal women be counseled about hormone therapy. While there was not enough evidence to recommend HT for all postmenopausal women, the Task Force advised that all women should discuss potential risks and benefits, and consider its use. That was then, this is now; we have new research information and can make more informed decisions about symptom management.

And the controversy continues. In 2004, researchers reanalyzed results from 30 other studies and concluded that benefits of HT outweigh risks when HT is started in women who have entered menopause recently. In this analysis, the risk of death was reduced, and HT was linked to helping prevent and possibly stop heart disease in women who had just entered menopause. The results also showed no change in the risk of death from breast cancer or other cancers, and a decreased risk for diabetes or breaking a hip. A new study is planned to provide even more information about the

Vasomotor symptoms

symptoms resulting from irregular function of the part of the brain that controls body heat, usually experienced as hot flashes and sweats that may or may not be followed by feeling cold or chilled.

use of hormones in women who are having moderate to severe symptoms and are just entering menopause.

There are no easy answers, but new information is continually becoming available that will shed more light on the risks and benefits for using hormone therapy.

Bridget's comment:

People tell me just to take my hormones and be quiet. Actually, I did for almost two years, and they're right. Hormones work like a charm. But I don't like taking them. They make me uneasy. In fact, I have a hunch that decreased estrogen is somehow linked to increased wisdom. I was counting on a little more wisdom in middle age. Or, to be more concrete, suppose a breast cancer connection pans out in the next few years. I worry about these things. Why take hormones that eradicate Saharan sex and make you feel and look like a 25-year-old when you can age naturally and develop wrinkles, heart disease, and osteoporosis? I grew a bra size on estrogen and felt like a foreigner in my own body. I didn't like it one bit. My gynecologist sympathizes with my predicament. He tells me all the pros and cons and latest study data on hormone therapy. Still, the ultimate decision is mine, and I've decided to face middle-age head-on. I stopped my hormones last month. The flash-filled days and nights are back with a vengeance. Wisdom is nowhere in sight.

82. What symptoms should I call to report when I am taking HT?

You should call your clinician if you have questions, are having bothersome side effects, or experience new symptoms after beginning HT. Sometimes a different regimen or type of estrogen or progestin will stop the bothersome side effects. And new symptoms could indicate health problems or reactions to the hormones. It's also important for you to call if you have any of the following symptoms, as they could point toward a serious reaction to HT. Although these are extremely rare, they should be reported to your clinician immediately:

- Abdominal pain, tenderness, or swelling
- Unexpected vaginal bleeding
- Breast lumps
- Coughing up blood
- Pain in your chest or calves
- Severe headache, dizziness, or faintness
- Sudden shortness of breath
- Vision changes
- Yellowing of the skin

83. How can I manage the side effects from the hormones so that I don't have to stop taking them?

If you are having side effects from taking HT, there are some specific lifestyle changes you can make to decrease the side effects. You also cannot assume that new symptoms—for example, headaches—are necessarily related to HT. You should discuss new symptoms or side effects with your clinician so they can be evaluated and treated if unrelated, or changes in the dose or type of estrogen or progesterone you are taking can be made, if appropriate. See Table 14 for managing the side effects of ET and EPT.

Table 14   Managing the Side Effects of ET or EPT

Side Effect	Management Suggestions
Abdominal bloating or cramps	• Do not eat grapefruit or drink grapefruit juice • Drink 6 to 8 glasses of water per day • Discuss with clinician reducing dose of progestin or taking a mild diuretic • Decrease salt intake
Breast changes or pain	• Wear supportive bra • Decrease chocolate, salt, peanuts, and caffeine • Discuss with your clinician reducing estrogen dose or changing the progestin • Consider evening primrose oil
Dry eyes or contact lens intolerance	• Use lubricating drops (made for contact lenses if appropriate) • Decrease wearing time of contacts • Discuss with eye care professional a change in the lenses you are wearing • Avoid cigarette smoke • Avoid antihistamines—they may make your eyes more dry and itchy
High blood pressure	• Take prescribed blood pressure medication • Monitor your blood pressure and report consistent elevations to your clinician • Exercise and maintain active lifestyle • Reduce salt intake • Lose weight if BMI >25 • Drink adequate fluids • Avoid alcohol and smoking
Fluid retention	• Reduce salt intake • Drink 6 to 8 glasses of water per day • Exercise • Discuss with your clinician changing from oral ET to an estrogen patch, cream, or gel; or reducing dose of progesterone; or changing to a different progesterone
Glucose intolerance or high blood sugars	• Discuss with your clinician how to adjust your insulin or oral diabetes medication • Follow your diet carefully • Exercise regularly • Discuss with your clinician reducing your estrogen dose

Table 14   Managing the Side Effects of ET or EPT (continued)

Side Effect	Management Suggestions
Hair loss on head or hair increase on body	• Discuss with your clinician changing to a different estrogen or progestin • Laser hair treatments for hair growth
Headache or migraine aggravation	• Drink 6 to 8 glasses of water per day • Decrease chocolate, salt, and alcohol • Discuss with your clinician changing to continuous-combined EPT or to transdermal ET, or change progestin dose • Avoid usual migraine triggers • Try magnesium supplements
Libido changes	• Change sexual routine • Discuss with clinician adding testosterone or replacing with different testosterone if already prescribed • Go out on a date • Spend time rekindling the romance in your relationship
Mood changes	• Decrease salt, caffeine, and alcohol • Discuss with clinician changing to different progestin or to continuous-combined EPT • Be sure you are getting enough sleep • Pay attention to stress management
Nausea and vomiting	• Take hormones with meals • Drink 6 to 8 glasses of water per day • Discuss with your clinician changing to transdermal estrogen, changing progestin type, or reducing dosages
Skin changes (dark patches), rash	• Always wear sunscreen, wear hat to shield face • If using patch, try a different location if adhesive causing the rash • If you develop hives, stop taking until you contact your clinician • Always make sure skin is clean and dry before applying patch
Vaginal bleeding/ spotting	• Be patient—breakthrough bleeding is common during the first few months of EPT • Take ET or EPT at the same time every day with food • Discuss with your clinician changing dose or type of HT if you cannot tolerate bleeding

Table 14   Managing the Side Effects of ET or EPT (continued)

Side Effect	Management Suggestions
Vaginal yeast infection	• Don't wear tight jeans • Reduce simple sugars in your diet • Keep vagina lubricated and moisturized
Vision changes	• Blurry vision and sudden decrease in vision or fields of vision are not acceptable side effects—contact your clinician immediately • Estrogen can change the shape of your cornea making contact lenses more difficult to fit
Weight changes*	• Maintain/develop a healthy diet • Drink 6 to 8 glasses of water per day • Daily calorie intake must be lowered at midlife to maintain same weight

*A study done in 1997 showed that women taking HT gained less weight than women not taking it.

Women taking HT actually gain less than women not taking it.

There is a longstanding belief that birth control pills and HT cause weight gain. But women taking HT actually gain less than women not taking it. Perhaps the reason women perceive that their weight gain is associated with HT is that HT helps them feel better, and they have a better appetite. More than likely, though, it is just the coincidence of time. Most women do add a few pounds at midlife.

84. How long can I be on estrogen therapy? My menopause started when I was 39. I'm now 52. If I need to stop the therapy, how do I do that?

It's very difficult to say how long you should stay on estrogen therapy if you have been on it for 13 years. If you started HT at a younger age due to medical reasons or premature menopause, then you might be advised to stay on it so that your body has the beneficial effects of those hormones until closer to the time of usual menopause. The current recommendation for women who experienced natural menopause is to use the lowest effective dose for the shortest possible period of time. We do have evidence from the WHI study that estrogen-progestin therapy (EPT) is safe for up to 5 years, and estrogen-only therapy (ET) for up to 6 years or more. After that, your risk for breast cancer increases by a small percentage. The WHI results also showed that risks for heart disease and stroke increase with 5 or 6 years of use. For women who continue to have moderate to severe menopausal symptoms, ET (or EPT if you have a uterus) is still the most effective treatment. You need to evaluate your quality of life, decide your tolerance for the symptoms, and make an informed decision based on having all of the information on the risks of HT available to you. If you are going to lie awake at night worrying whether you're going to get breast cancer or have a stroke, there is little point in staying on hormone therapy. If, on the other hand, you cannot tolerate the return of sleepless nights and drenching hot flashes, HT's benefits may outweigh the potential risks.

There is little guidance available to clinicians about stopping hormone therapy. Many women who stopped taking EPT "cold-turkey" after hearing about the WHI study results reported that they had a return of their symptoms, and in some cases, their symptoms came back worse than ever. As a result, most clinicians now recommend that women wean off HT in tapering doses over a long period of time. Tapering can be done in several ways. It might mean alternating your usual dose with a lower dose every other day for a week, and then taking the lower dose consistently for several weeks. Or, if you are already on the lowest dose, tapering might mean skipping a dose 1 or 2 days a week. Tapering doses over a period of weeks helps your body to gradually become accustomed to lower levels of the hormones. This, in turn, may keep you from developing rebound symptoms such as hot flashes or breakthrough bleeding. Breakthrough bleeding is not a common effect from tapering off HT, but if it occurs, it should be discussed with your clinician. Tapering is an issue that you should discuss with your clinician every year. The goal is always to get acceptable relief from your symptoms on the lowest dose of the hormones.

It's probably a good idea to reduce the dosage once every year or two to see how your symptoms are doing. Whenever hormones get bad press, some women quit "cold turkey." This can make your symptoms reappear and may even make them worse than they were before you took HT to begin with. If you've decided that you can't tolerate being off the hormones, it's a good idea to go back to your previous dose until the symptoms subside, and then start lowering the dose slowly (as described above) to see if you can either reduce your dose or wean yourself off. Of course, it's always advisable to call your clinician before you make any changes.

85. What are natural hormones? How are they different from the estrogen and progesterone that I have been taking to control my symptoms?

"Natural" is a confusing term when applied to hormones. "Natural" products are those whose major component is derived from animal, plant, or mineral sources. This does not mean that a substance is bio-identical (short for "biologically identical"), which means that the substance has the exact same chemical structure as that found in the human body. For example, the prescription form of estrogen that is made from pregnant mare's urine (Premarin®) could be considered natural because it is made from an animal source. However, it's not bio-identical to the estrogens that a woman's body makes. When a woman asks for natural hormones, she is more than likely asking for bio-identical hormones.

Bio-identical hormones include 17-beta-estradiol, estrone, estriol, progesterone, testosterone, and DHEA, and are extracted from soybean and Mexican wild yam, an herb. Bio-identical hormones are chemically synthesized in a laboratory using the plant sources. Women cannot just eat wild yam and lots of soy to get the same effects. Women's bodies can absorb the hormones that are extracted from yam and soy and chemically synthesized in the laboratory, but their bodies cannot change the yam and soy molecules into bio-identical hormones.

DHEA is available as a dietary supplement. It is usually a single-ingredient product, but is also found in products with other herbals. DHEA is converted to testosterone in the body and is sometimes used to manage low libido (see Questions 67 about DHEA and low libido).

All hormone preparations, bio-identical or not, carry risks and benefits. All hormones that are taken by mouth are processed in the liver. Some speculate that bio-identical hormones are better for the liver than other hormones. But there is no scientific evidence to support this claim. Even though bio-identical hormones are chemically the same as those produced in the body, when they are taken as therapy rather than produced by the body itself, they carry risks. The FDA requires *all* prescription hormones, including bio-identical hormones, to carry the same warnings on their labels.

86. Can I get natural (bio-identical) hormones over the counter (OTC), or do I need a prescription? Are natural hormones safe to take? If natural hormones can be made from soy, would I get the same effect if I just eat more soy or soybean products?

Often, when women are seeking natural hormones, they are interested in "bio-identical" hormones, or hormones that are chemically the same as those produced by the body. With the exception of a few progesterone creams, bio-identical hormones must be prescribed by a clinician. If you and your clinician decide that bio-identical hormones would be best for you, several preparations are available from regular or compounding pharmacies. Compounding pharmacists can combine bio-identical hormones (estradiol, estriol, estrone, progesterone, and testosterone) with the appropriate base substance, such as vegetable oil, to create oral forms like capsules or drops that are placed under the tongue (**sublingual**) in the exact dosage prescribed by your clinician. Compounding pharmacists can also make topical creams and gels that are applied to the skin or vagina. Several regular pharmacies also com-

Sublingual
under the tongue.

pound hormone prescriptions. Check with your local pharmacy to find out if there is a registered pharmacist on staff who can compound your bio-identical hormone prescription for you.

There are a number of over-the-counter progesterone creams. However, the exact dosage of the progesterone portion of the cream is not always available on the label. Dosages may vary from 2 to 700 mg per ounce. Creams are used on the skin or vagina, usually twice a day. The application may be simple, but it's not so easy to determine the number of milligrams actually absorbed. Although **injectable** and oral forms of progestins have been shown to ease hot flashes for some women (see Question 77 about using PT for hot flashes), whether creams or gels work for hot flashes is less clear. Progesterone creams do not seem to provide enough hormones to prevent overgrowth of the uterine lining. If you want to try a progesterone cream to control your symptoms, it is best to have one prescribed and compounded for you with a specific number of milligrams.

If women are using "natural" (bio-identical) nonprescription hormones, they are often under the assumption that the hormones are also safe. But the FDA does not regulate nonprescription and some compounded pharmacy hormones like they do prescription medicines. And remember that all hormones, including bio-identical hormones, have potential side effects and risks.

The biggest challenge in comparing the safety of some bio-identical hormones is that there have been few scientific studies evaluating their effects or comparing them with traditional hormones. So, we don't

Injectable
given into the muscle or fat tissue using a needle with a syringe attached.

know how they stack up to each other. For example, we don't know if bio-identical hormones prevent bone loss as Premarin® does. Women who want menopause symptom relief need to understand that bio-identical hormones may carry the same risks to health as other hormone preparations that are not chemically identical to those produced in the body. As with any medication or therapy to alleviate your menopausal symptoms, your clinician should review with you all of the potential risks and benefits currently known.

Your body is not able to change wild yam or soy into estrogen or progesterone. So there's no point in trying to get the natural hormones by eating Mexican wild yam or lots of soy. Soy does have some other benefits, though, so adding it to your diet is still a good idea.

87. My healthcare provider wants to prescribe Prozac for my hot flashes. Is it okay to take an antidepressant for that reason?

Yes. Antidepressants like Effexor®, Zoloft®, Prozac®, and Paxil® have shown promising results when used for hot flashes. Some women are already taking Prozac® or Serefem® (fluoxetine) for some form of depression. A "side effect" from taking these medicines is a reduction in hot flashes. It is not yet clear if the severe mood changes associated with premenstrual depression are caused by high levels of progesterone or by low levels of estrogen. If the latter is true, mood symptoms may get even worse when the low estrogen levels of menopause occur. If you are already on an antidepressant for severe premenstrual moods, you should not stop taking it when you have stopped having your periods for a year. Many medications, including antidepressants, must be stopped slowly to avoid withdrawal symptoms, which, in some cases, can be very severe and unpleasant.

Some antidepressants can cause sexual side effects such as inability or difficulty reaching orgasm, and lack of libido. For postmenopausal women who are already experiencing sexual problems due to urinary or genital changes and discomfort during intercourse, antidepressants with sexual side effects may not be a good choice for managing hot flashes.

It usually takes several weeks for antidepressants to have an effect on depression, but when they are taken for hot flashes, the response can be almost immediate to a couple of weeks. Side effects are common in the early weeks of treatment, but may disappear with time.

See Table 15 for considerations and side effects of the most common antidepressants prescribed for hot flashes.

88. What other prescription medications can be used for hot flashes?

For women who prefer to avoid or can't take HT, there are other prescription medicines that can provide some relief from hot flashes. These medications have other primary reasons for being prescribed, but do offer another option to women besides HT or alternative therapies.

Neurontin® (gabapentin), usually used for seizures or chronic pain management, can help with hot flashes in

Table 15   Non-Hormone Prescription Medications for Hot Flashes

Type of Medication	Name	Comments
Depression Medications	venlafaxine (Effexor)	• Usually works right away for hot flashes, less quickly for depression • Can interact with other medications, St. John's wort, or valerian • Reduce dosage gradually when discontinuing • Can cause poor appetite, nausea, vomiting, mouth dryness
	fluoxetine (Prozac)	• Usually works right away for hot flashes, less quickly for depression • Can interact with other medications, e.g., St. John's wort • Reduce dosage gradually when discontinuing • Can cause nausea, sweating, fatigue, weakness, poor libido, difficulty with orgasm
	paroxetine (Paxil)	• Same considerations and side effects as Prozac • Reduce dosage gradually when discontinuing
Seizure medications	gabapentin (Neurontin)	• Avoid antacids within 2 hours of use • Can cause tiredness, loss of balance, dizziness
Blood pressure medications	clonidine (Catapres)	• Reduce dose gradually when discontinuing • Also available as a patch • Can cause constipation, rash, dry mouth, nausea, tiredness, dizziness, weakness, sleeplessness, muscle aches, agitation, low blood pressure, irregular heartbeat • Less effective than depression medicines, more effective than gabapentin

doses as low as 100 mg/day. The amount of medication is slowly increased up to 900 mg/day until hot flashes are reduced. The most common adverse effects are usually found when higher doses are used to treat seizure disorders (3,000 to 3,600 mg/day), including sleepiness, abnormal eye movements, dizziness, tiredness, and loss of balance. The biggest problem for women is that Neurontin® (gabapentin) is very sedating, so it's better tolerated when taken at bedtime. Sometimes the feelings of fatigue can carry over into the next day.

Although Catapres® (clonidine) is used for high blood pressure and can have some important side effects, including nausea, fatigue, dizziness, and dry mouth, hot flashes can be reduced substantially, especially when the clonidine patch is used. Other adverse effects from clonidine include very slow heart rate, low blood pressure, and irregular heart rhythms.

Megace® (megestrol) is a progestin-based medication that is usually used in the treatment of advanced cancers of the breast or uterine lining, but can be helpful in the treatment of hot flashes when used in much smaller doses. Side effects include stomach upset, weight gain, chest pain, fluid retention, high blood pressure, high blood sugar levels, rash, fever, difficulty sleeping, urinary frequency, weakness, decreased sex drive, and indigestion. It should be used with caution if you have diabetes or have had a blood clot.

89. I've heard that androgens such as testosterone will help my lack of sex drive. Is that true?

Libido, or sex drive, is more highly linked with androgens (especially testosterone) than with estrogen. The only FDA-approved medicines for women that contain testosterone are Estratest®, Estratest HS®, Syntest®, and Menogen®, which are combination pills of estrogen and testosterone. These preparations are approved for a cyclic regimen (3 weeks on, 1 week off), but many clinicians prescribe them for continuous daily use. A progestin is needed if you have a uterus because androgens, in this case testosterone, do not provide protection for the uterine lining. The only FDA-approved indication for taking estrogen-testosterone combination pills is moderate to severe hot flashes and sweats not relieved by other forms of estrogen. Even though not FDA-approved for the treatment of women with sexual dysfunction, many clinicians do prescribe them for that reason.

Almost half of testosterone is processed out by the liver before it gets into the bloodstream, so larger doses of testosterone have to be taken by women in order to get the desired effect. Only about 2% of testosterone in the blood is free to be used by the body. Your body needs that 2% of testosterone in order to have a normal sex drive.

Although a testosterone and estrogen injection (Climacteron®) is available in Canada, it is not currently available in the United States. The FDA has not approved it due to concerns about the elevated testosterone levels that may result. Depo-Testadiol® (estrogen and testosterone mixture) is available in the United States as a monthly injection for the treatment of moderate to severe hot flashes and sweats.

Testosterone cream or ointment (2%) can be applied to the genitals or any skin surface. Some women report improvement in their sex drive using the cream or ointment. It is usually prescribed ⅛ to ¼ teaspoon applied twice a day. Testosterone gels and patches that are available are not recommended for women because they are manufactured to treat testosterone deficiency in men and contain too much testosterone for women. A new testosterone patch, designed for women, is currently being evaluated, so a new option may be available in the future.

The safety of staying on any form of androgen therapy for longer than 2 years is unknown.

The important adverse reactions to estrogen-testosterone preparations are the same as for estrogens, but also include a rare form of liver inflammation (hepatitis) and liver cancer. The most common side effects of testosterone are developing male characteristics, which include acne, deepened voice, enlargement of the clitoris, male pattern baldness or thinning of hair, lowering of the good cholesterol (HDL), and weight gain (especially in the abdomen). Side effects don't usually happen if testosterone levels are kept in the normal range. You may also experience estrogen-related side effects because testosterone is converted to estrogen in the body. Testosterone can cause mood elevation because of its beneficial effect on serotonin. And, for this reason, testosterone can be addicting. Testosterone treatment should be used with great caution in women with diabetes because of its effect on glucose.

Viagra® (sildenafil), which is used in men with **erectile dysfunction**, has been evaluated for use in women and was found not to be effective. It's no surprise that women require more than just a pill to improve sex for them. But other medications used for sexual problems in men are also being tested for possible use in women—so there may be more options in the future.

Erectile dysfunction
inability to make the penis rigid.

Ginny's comment:

I really love my husband, I do. He's my best friend too—but I just had no interest in sex. Now that I am using the testosterone I feel like a different woman. It isn't perfect—but it has made a very positive difference for me.

90. Are there medical treatments or medications that are used to treat urinary incontinence?

There are many options for women with urge and stress incontinence. If you have tried the alternative therapies and lifestyle changes described in Question 68 without relief, prescription medications or surgery may be helpful for you. The main thing is not to suffer in silence. Urinary incontinence is not uncommon and can be managed successfully in most cases.

The FemSoft Insert® is a tiny silicone tube that acts as a stopper when the woman inserts it into her urethra during a visit to the bathroom. Each silicone insert is used only one time and then discarded; a new one is inserted after each bathroom visit. FemSoft® is available only by prescription and is very effective against stress incontinence. It has been successfully tested in women who experience exercise-induced incontinence.

Vaginal dryness experienced in postmenopause can make urinary incontinence worse. Treating the changes with vaginal estrogen cream or ring can be very helpful in lessening incontinence. It can take several weeks to get a full effect, but some women notice a difference after only a few days. There isn't a good answer about how long local estrogen therapy can be used. Many clinicians recommend using the least amount of vaginal estrogen cream needed to get an acceptable benefit.

Medications for urge incontinence include:

- Anticholinergics: A group of medications that reduce incontinence by causing urine retention and reducing bladder spasms. Ditropan® (oxybutynin) comes in pill and patch forms. The side effects of anticholinergic drugs include dry mouth, sleepiness, and urine retention. In this case, urine retention is the intended effect. Constipation is another side effect, but because straining at stool contributes to urinary incontinence, this is not a good side effect. If you want to continue on an anticholingergic for your incontinence, it's important to increase the fiber in your diet (prunes, prune juice, raisins, vegetables, fruits, and whole grains), moderately increase water, and avoid white rice and bananas, which tend to be constipating. Detrol® (tolterodine) has similar effects as Ditropan®, but in some women causes less dry mouth. Sanctura® (trospium chloride) is a new medication that was recently approved by the FDA for the treatment of overactive bladder and urinary incontinence. The most common side effects include dry mouth and constipation.
- Tricyclic antidepressants, such as Tofranil® (imipramine), can be useful for urge incontinence in women who also have depression or chronic pain. Imipramine works because it has anticholinergic side effects and can cause urine retention. Imipramine is one of the few drugs that has been found to be effective against both urge and stress incontinence.
- Bentyl® (dicyclomine) is an antispasm drug usually used in the treatment of irritable bowel syndrome (IBS). It also has anticholinergic effects, which can be helpful in the treatment of urge incontinence.

- Local estrogen therapy in the form of vaginal rings, suppositories, or creams is more effective than the oral, gel, or patch forms of estrogen for urinary incontinence. A combination of Sudafed® (pseudoephedrine) and vaginal estrogen cream can be effective in the treatment of urge incontinence. Vaginal estrogen in combination with oxybutynin or imipramine has helped stress incontinence. There has been some recent evidence that using oral EPT (estrogen-progestin therapy) might increase urinary incontinence.

Surgery for urge incontinence is rarely done due to the complications associated with it. The use of medications should be tried if behavioral methods for the management of incontinence don't work (see Question 68 regarding behavioral methods for managing incontinence). Surgery should be considered only as a last resort for urge incontinence. A surgically implanted device intended to stimulate the sacral nerve has been effective in some women who have not responded to lifestyle changes and medications for urge incontinence.

Surgery for stress incontinence is more common but is usually reserved for when Kegel exercises and medicines have been unsuccessful. Most surgeries involve making a sling or suturing the vaginal wall to support the bladder and take pressure off the muscles supporting the bladder. This surgery is called a **TVT (trans-vaginal tuck)** and is usually done with conscious sedation in an operating room. You will not be allowed to go home until you have been able to urinate.

There are more simple surgical procedures that are also being used. One involves the use of fat that is taken from some other area in your body or collagen, which

TVT (trans-vaginal tuck)

stands for trans-vaginal-tuck, a surgical procedure in which some tissue is made into a sling-type arrangement that supports the bladder and urethra in the treatment of stress incontinence.

is injected to support the urethra. Another procedure, called Gynecare TVT (tension-free vaginal tape), can be done using a local or regional anesthetic. An incision is made in the vagina and a mesh ribbon-like tape is threaded through the incision behind the urethra to the outside of the body in the pubic area. The ribbon provides support for the urethra, reducing leakage of urine. The procedure usually takes no more than 30 minutes. The patient is asked to cough to make sure the ribbon is at the proper tension to prevent urine leakage. The ribbon is then snipped below the skin and sewn in place.

Sarah's comment:

One of the things that bugged me the most was the "water works." So embarrassing and depressing! Doing the vaginal/abdominal exercises didn't work. I finally had a long talk with my doctor and she recommended a GYN/urologist—"my savior." I ended up having the sling procedure. A series of diagnostic tests to be sure this would be helpful, then a quick 4-hour outpatient visit, and then a miracle— after less than a week, no more "leaks" or uncontrollable urgency. Only downfall or precaution was no lifting over 8 pounds for 8 weeks—and one of my cats weighs 20 pounds! It's now been over a year and so far, so good.

PART SIX

Menopause: You and Your Family

In some ways, I want to change my life. Is that a common feeling during menopause?

Some people say that women become more creative during menopause. Is that true?

Is it normal to mourn the loss of my fertility?

How can I help my partner understand what I'm going through?

More ...

91. How do women perceive menopause?

Menopause is far more than symptoms and an end to monthly periods.

Menopause is far more than symptoms and an end to monthly periods. Menopause, for any woman, is going to be defined not only by what symptoms she experiences, but also by her expectations, emotions, and relationships.

Menopause is a normal life transition in spite of negative symptoms. Many women view menopause as the change from a reproductive stage to a nonreproductive stage, and recognize their changing health risks and needs. Society may have a more negative view as they see women change from being young and fertile to being older and unable to reproduce. But most women who are experiencing menopause say it is fine, it is a normal part of life, and that society needs to have a new perspective. This double standard can make it awkward for women who don't feel they need to take things for their hot flashes, but who also don't want to have hot flashes in public because they are concerned about how others will see them—they don't want to be labeled as "old."

Many women see menopause as a time to take stock in their lives and make changes for better health. Some women view menopause as a time when they can concentrate on themselves, like losing the weight they've been carrying around for too long. They become more concerned about their health, and start making the lifestyle changes that they have been putting off for years, like exercising, stopping smoking, and having a better diet. They use this time as an opportunity to reassess not only their health, but also their relationships and other areas of their lives.

Whatever your viewpoint, it is important to stay as positive as you can. Having a good attitude can improve your health; in fact, being negative has been linked with higher death rates and more illnesses! So, remember that menopause is a normal part of life and that the symptoms will decrease with time. Keep your chin up, stand up for yourself, and find something to feel good about every day.

Having a good attitude can improve your health.

Felicia's comment:

I've taken it all of my life. Now I'm 50. I've lived through this much. If I need to say no, then I'm going to say no. I'm not going to spend a lot of energy worrying about whether the other person has misinterpreted my message. Of course I'll try to explain it to them, but at the end of the day, I've come this far and I've attained a certain status. I am going to be me, this is who I am—no more games, no more playing it their way, it's time for me, and I need to take care of myself for a change.

92. In some ways, I feel like I want to change my life. Is that a common feeling during menopause?

Many women find a new contentment with their lives when they reach menopause. Other women feel unsettled and want to make changes. Sometimes a bad marriage or partnership comes to an end or changes are made to make a relationship more fulfilling. Some women want to go back to work outside the home if they stopped their careers when they had children. Menopause can also be a time to develop new interests and new relationships.

Asking yourself some of the following questions may help you evaluate your current life circumstances:

- Is my family what I hoped for? Did I develop the kinds of relationships with my family that I wanted?
- How healthy and successful are my children?
- How satisfied do I feel with my partner? Am I satisfied being alone?
- Do I have the career that I envisioned for myself? Should I change careers?
- Have I been as successful as I hoped?
- Am I as healthy as I could be or hoped to be at this stage of my life?
- What kind of changes in my life would make me happier right now?
- Have I made the type of mark on the world that I hoped?

It's very common for both men and women to feel the need for change around midlife as a result of taking stock of their lives. They may experience a sense of loss, regret, or sadness if they have not accomplished or become what they had planned. If you don't feel good about the answers to the above questions, menopause may be time for you to make some changes.

93. Some people think that women become more creative during menopause. Is that true?

Certainly, some women do become more creative. But it's not like you wake up one morning after you reach menopause and decide that you're going to be creative. Instead, women often ask themselves, "How do I want to live this next phase of my life?" Because of this self-reflection, some women will put more energy into creative activities.

Menopause can be a time when you can spend more energy on the pastimes and hobbies that you may have given up to raise children or further your career. You may decide to take up a new hobby. You might even make a change to a career that is more fulfilling and allows more of your talents to shine.

Some speculate that the reason women become more creative after menopause is that they are refocusing their reproductive and nurturing roles that were previously channeled into giving birth and raising children, to a new area of their lives. On the other hand, it's not fair to build the expectation, "My hormones changed, now I'm creative."

94. Is it normal to mourn the loss of my fertility?

Yes, it's very normal. But not all women will experience the loss of fertility in the same way. In fact, many women rejoice in the fact that they can no longer get pregnant after menopause. This new freedom from the risk of pregnancy can make lovemaking more spontaneous.

Not all women will experience the loss of fertility in the same way.

Others, even though they do not actually want to birth another child, feel the loss of the ability to have a baby more acutely. These women may mourn not being able to raise any more children.

This feeling of loss may be most poignant in those who were never able to conceive but really wanted children. In fact, some women report that the single greatest upset related to menopause, including the discomfort of hot flashes, is the loss of their fertility.

Being sad about your loss of fertility is normal. However, persistent feelings of sadness may be a sign of depression, and you may need to discuss your feelings of loss with a mental health professional. See Question 41 about recognizing depression.

Debra's comment:

But I felt it, I felt less attractive. And it was like a void, no more like nostalgia—you know, when you see a new baby, one of those teeny weenie ones, and you know your body can't do that anymore. It took awhile to get over it. I wonder if a man will want me if I can't have babies—will he find me attractive, or am I just all over?

95. My body image is pretty bad. I feel old, fat, and wrinkled. How can I feel better about my appearance when I hit menopause?

Your breasts may be sagging, your middle increasing, and your teeth requiring more and more crowns, but you are a) not alone, and b) still able to reverse some of the signs of aging. It probably feels like the number of wrinkles, your waist circumference, and the number of gray hairs increased all at the same time. But they didn't, and it will take some work to lose some weight and tone your muscles.

It will take some work to lose some weight and tone your muscles.

Some women refuse to color their hair, instead preferring to let their gray hair show as a badge of honor. Others cover up the gray as fast as it appears. The same with wrinkles: some women feel they've earned every one, while others get Botox® injections every few months or seek plastic surgery to change their appearance.

Without estrogen, your skin will also lose its elasticity. Your face wrinkles will become more apparent, and your breasts and buttocks will sag. The fat around your waist, a common occurrence in midlife, is definitely something you can manage if you are willing to lose weight and exercise. See Question 61 for improving your diet, and Question 69 for exercise suggestions.

Skin ages fairly well when left to its own devices. If you smoke, your skin will wrinkle faster. Hydrated skin withstands aging better, so drink lots of water. Sun damage is the leading cause of wrinkles, not lack of hormones, so it's important to use a 15 to 30 SPF sunblock every time you go outside. Some dermatologists recommend hats and sunblock even when walking to your car from the house. Make sure to use sunblock on the easily forgotten places like the tips of your ears, the back of your neck, the backs of your hands, and your lips.

Even being out in the wind can dry out your skin. Believe it or not, the forces of gravity are still working as we age, gradually pulling our skin earthward, causing sagging and wrinkling. There is less collagen in the skin with aging, and the skin itself thins, making wrinkles more apparent. Brownish spots on your skin are related to sun exposure and not your changing hormones. HT may cause skin darkening (**melasma** or **chloasma**), especially if you don't use daily sunblock. The ratio of estrogen to androgen contributes to oil production in the skin, and some women develop adult acne when their hormones are chaotic. If you are taking testosterone to manage your hot flashes or other menopausal symptoms, you may also be more likely to develop acne. Using a moisturizer with sunblock is a good combination for skin protection. The B vitamins are also known

Melasma

patches of darkened skin that occur as a result of exposure to sun, aging, or as a side effect of medication.

Chloasma

patches of darkened skin that may result from aging, sun, or as a medication side effect.

to help keep skin hydrated and healthier looking. So, adding a vitamin B complex and using a moisturizer regularly may help keep skin moisturized and more elastic. Vitamin C creams (such as orange daily C serum or Cellex-C®) available without prescription or Vitamin A creams (such as Retin-A®) available by prescription may also help reduce the signs of aging.

Hair will change with age, and not just to gray or white. Hair can become drier, sometimes curlier or straighter, and the gray hairs can become more wiry and coarse. Avoid drying shampoos and hair products with alcohol. You may also develop some thinning on the crown of your head. Conversely, you may gain those rogue stiff chin hairs or fine peach-fuzz on your face. The changed estrogen-to-androgen ratio is also responsible for these hair changes. Hair texture changes and loss can also be due to thyroid disease, iron deficiency anemia, excessive dieting, sudden changes in hormones, intense stress, and Vitamin B_{12} deficiency. Talk to your clinician about adjusting hormone dosages to reduce hair loss or about medications that may be helpful in restoring hair growth.

You can remove unwanted hair with laser treatments (dark hair on fair skin responds best), depilatory creams (chemical reactions are common), shaving, or waxing. There is also a new prescription cream available called Vaniqa® (eflornithine), which reduces unwanted facial hair (hair will regrow when you stop using it).

Tooth loss is associated with osteoporosis. The faster women lose bone during postmenopause, the more likely they are to lose teeth—another good reason to prevent osteoporosis! There is some controversy about whether there is an association between bone loss and gum disease. Lower levels of estrogen are associated with inflammatory changes and thinning of the gum tissue, making you more susceptible to injury, infection, and tooth sensitivity. Some women have a burning sensation in the mouth and on the tongue during postmenopause, probably related to lower estrogen levels and unbound estrogen receptors in the mouth. The burning sensation can also be due to diabetes, infection, or certain types of anemia, so it's important to get that checked out. You should discuss how to protect your teeth and gums with your dental professional. Making sure you get enough calcium to prevent tooth loss is especially important. If you are concerned about the appearance of your teeth, cosmetic dentistry or whitening systems may be an option. But the ingredients in the whitening systems can be irritating to gum tissue that may already be inflamed for other reasons, although the irritation usually goes away with time.

The need for reading glasses is probably a fact of life for most women at menopause. If you wear glasses all of the time or if you just wear them for reading, have fun picking out something that makes a statement about you. Reading glasses don't have to make you look old.

Not only do many women have concerns about how they look at midlife, but body odors can be a cause for concern as well. Some women experience increased body odor from sweats or vaginal discharge. Using perfume or showering with perfumed soap may reduce the odor from sweating, but many of these products can be drying to the skin. Using antiperspirants that also contain deodorants can be helpful. Scented moisturizers might be helpful as long as they are not applied to the genital areas where perfumes can be very irritating, and may actually make the problem worse. Douching should be avoided. It will not reduce vaginal discharge. Douching disrupts the natural bacteria of the vagina and is likely to increase discharge because the body will try to reestablish the normal bacteria balance. Sparing use of plain, unscented cornstarch may help to absorb some perspiration and odor, and dressing in breathable fabrics and avoiding the use of nylon stockings can be helpful, too.

Menopause is really an excellent time to reevaluate your lifestyle and how it relates to your appearance. If you are overweight and feeling uncomfortable with your appearance, it's a good time to start eating more healthy foods and exercising. Cutting down on alcohol and stopping cigarette smoking are two good places to start in developing a healthier lifestyle. Avoiding alcohol and cigarettes will improve your skin appearance and overall health. If you exercise, you may have fewer symptoms and get better sleep, giving you a more rested appearance.

Trina's comment:

I'm taking charge here. I'm going to concentrate on getting myself healthy, like losing the weight. I am going to eat better and get exercise. Today is the first day of the rest of my life, and I am going to be here to live it to the fullest!

96. How can I help my partner understand what I'm going through?

While it may sound trite for women who have been around long enough to experience menopause, honesty is still the best policy. Honest communication will help your partner, female or male, to understand what you're going through. If your partner is female, she may be experiencing her own menopausal symptoms. If your partner is male, he may have his own version of menopause, called "**andropause**," and be experiencing similar symptoms such as poor sleep, irritability, and sexual problems.

Tell your partner what's going on. Share this book. Sign up together for the online newsletter, Menopause Flashes, from the North American Menopause Society (*www.nams.org*). Most mothers have not traditionally shared their menopause experiences with their children, and menopause isn't frequently discussed in social situations, so your partner may really be in the dark. Many women feel that there is still a social taboo around talking about menopause, whether it's with other women or with their families.

Your partner may be misunderstanding your negative moods and actions. The more you share, the more your partner can understand that you are going through a natural phase of life, but that the symptoms can feel anything but natural to you. You may display behavior that makes it appear that you are rejecting your partner when, in fact, your hormones are in chaos. If you are having a cranky kind of day, tell your partner that you're having a bad hormone day and it's not the partner's fault. The more you keep to yourself, the more likely it is that anger and conflict will erupt between you and your partner.

Let your partner help you. And tell him or her what you need. If you need to sleep with the window open and the fan to be more comfortable at night, tell your partner. It's an important time for understanding and compromise.

Andropause

short for androgenpause. Applied to men, it's a period of time that is speculated to be similar to menopause in women; a time of shifting hormones and midlife changes.

251

If you are withdrawing from sex with your partner because you have no interest or you're worried about the discomfort caused by vaginal dryness, your partner may think you've lost interest in him or her. Keep the lines of communication going. Tell your partner what might make sex more pleasurable for you. Make a date night, go out and have some quiet time to talk about some of the changes you both are experiencing. See Questions 66, 67, and 89 about ways to help vaginal dryness and the lack of sex drive.

Partners of women experiencing menopause can find all of the changes confusing and maybe even threatening. It can seem like the person they partnered with has changed into someone they don't really recognize or understand anymore. Swings in emotions and reduced patience can change how you respond to comments or even jokes that you have shared with your partner for years. Symptoms may seem unbelievable to your partner, leaving you feeling like they think you are kidding or even making it up. This can cause added stress to both of you and in your relationship together.

Midlife and menopause can be a time of stressful changes. Some women decide at midlife that they are tired of abusive relationships with partners. Don't be a victim. If you need help getting out of an abusive relationship, it's important to talk with your clinician and use the resources you're offered to separate from an abuser. You don't have to wait to be asked by your clinician if you are being threatened physically or verbally. Please see Question 100 about where to go for more information on domestic violence and for all aspects of menopause.

Menopause can be an opportunity for positive change. While you may be making some positive health changes, your partner might benefit from the same changes. Take up walking together. Start drinking decaffeinated coffee together. Make a commitment together to eat a healthy diet.

There's no clear recipe for helping your partner understand what you're going through. Each woman's experience is different, and each partner's response to her experience is different, too. Some partners "get it" and seem to know instinctively what to do. Others need step-by-step instructions on how to help you. You need the support of a loving partner at this time in your life. Ask for help and support if you are not receiving it.

Diana's comment:

My husband, he doesn't understand why I keep the air on... he doesn't understand that, he thinks I just want to run the bill up, how do you like that? And you know what? I don't even bother keeping it going through the motions to explain it to him because he's thinking I'm making it up. Here I am, sweat pouring off my face, and he thinks I'm just making it up to annoy him and keep the air on. And that's another part of stress, when you and your mate don't get along and you're not feeling well, all those things play a key role because when you don't feel well, he should be able to understand and take good care of you. Even if he doesn't understand you, he should be able to empathize.

97. I've recently heard that men go through their own version of menopause. Is that true?

There doesn't seem to be a point in time when men experience a definitive drop in their testosterone levels, even though their testosterone levels will diminish over time as they age. Men can father children into their 80s and do not abruptly lose their fertility the same way women do.

There is a phenomenon among men at midlife, sometimes called "andropause." Some studies have indicated that men experience many changes at midlife such as memory changes, fatigue, sleep changes, vision changes, sexual changes, and moodiness. These are the same changes that women experience during perimenopause and after, which begs the question, "Are midlife changes related to hormones, or just to the aging process?"

Men are more at risk for sexual dysfunction and heart disease as they age. They are more apt to put on weight, particularly around their stomachs. The risk for osteoporosis increases as men age, but they are not at the same high risk for it as women are.

So, when you're experiencing the symptoms of menopause, the man in your life may be experiencing many similar symptoms. When you're both having symptoms, this increases the possibility of conflict between the two of you. Letting your partner know what you're going through and listening to him about his symptoms will make coping with menopause and andropause easier for both of you.

98. What should I tell my children about menopause?

Honest communication is as important with your children as it is with your spouse or partner. Obviously, discussions with children need to be age-appropriate.

Most older school-aged children and adolescents are old enough to understand hot flashes and mood swings. Explain what menopause is, how it makes you feel sometimes, and ask for their understanding about some of the symptoms that may be there one day and gone the next. Relate what you're feeling to what they may be going through. For example, when they've stayed up late doing homework and they don't want to get up to go to school, they may be irritable from lack of sleep. Relate their experience of not getting a good night's sleep to yours. Reassure them that you're not ill. Younger children particularly may think you are sick, especially when you involuntarily reach for your chest during a hot flash and start sweating. Also, reassure children that you are not angry with them when you are feeling irritable. It is important to discuss how you feel so that children do not erroneously think they are causing your distress, even though you may be feeling less patient with their behavior.

You can explain that there are a lot of hormone changes and that menopause marks the end of fertility. You can add that these hormone changes bring on a variety of symptoms, including hot flashes, forgetfulness, irritability, and sometimes depression. Your children need to know that they are not causing the symptoms, and that they can help you cope better by being cooperative and understanding. It's probably not necessary to discuss vaginal dryness and changes in libido, unless your child is an adult female, and then it might be beneficial for her to learn about how you are coping with these normal changes.

Conveying what you're going through is as important for sons as it is for daughters. Your daughters will eventually go through menopause, and your sons may have a partner some day who is going through it. Give them a good idea of how menopause has affected you and how you try to cope with the symptoms. Once they know the nature of your menopause experience, they'll know that they need to put on a sweater when you open a window in freezing weather, rather than think you're trying to freeze them out. Having a sense of humor when it comes to menopause can help the whole family cope with unpleasant symptoms.

Having a sense of humor when it comes to menopause can help the whole family cope with unpleasant symptoms.

99. I work with a lot of younger people. They will occasionally make remarks about my hot flashes and getting older. What should I say to them?

Those young people and many others have been sold a bill of goods by the media—that menopause means you're getting old and dried up. The baby-boomer generation is smack in the middle of perimenopause and menopause, and they have an opportunity to make aging look pretty good to the younger folks.

When someone makes a remark to you about hot flashes or your age because you're "menopausal," you need to respond to the extent that you're comfortable. Wishing the same miserable symptoms on the young person doesn't educate them. You can be direct with them about several things. First, menopause is a natural transition in midlife just like puberty was a transition when they were younger. Second, there may be symptoms related to hormone changes that you have no control over. There are treatments for these symptoms but sometimes the treatments don't work. Tell the young person that you are very uncomfortable when you have a hot flash and there's very little way to disguise it, and that some women feel that their hot flashes announce to everyone that they are going through menopause and are getting older. And lastly, there are some real advantages to getting older—more freedom, more control over money and health, and an opportunity to make aging a positive experience.

100. Where do I go for more information about menopause?

It can be gratifying to share your experiences with other women. It's also helpful to hear from women who have learned healthy ways of coping with menopause. If you want to do some research on your own before discussing symptoms, lifestyle changes, and options for treatment with your clinician, the organizations, resources, and web sites in Appendix A might be helpful to you.

Appendix A

Menopause and Women's Health

American College of Nurse-Midwives
818 Connecticut Avenue NW, Suite 900
Washington, DC 20006
(202) 728-9860
www.midwife.org

American College of Obstetricians and Gynecologists
409 12th St., SW, PO Box 96920
Washington, DC 20090-6920
(202) 863-2518 (patient information brochures)
www.acog.org

**Clinical Trials: A Service of the National Institutes of Health
(linking patients to medical research)**
www.clinicaltrials.gov

Early Menopause.com
www.earlymenopause.com

National Association of Nurse Practitioners in Women's Health
503 Capitol Court, NE, Suite 300
Washington, DC 20002
(202) 543-9693
www.npwh.org

National Women's Health Information Center
United States Department of Health and Human Services
(800) 994-9662
www.4women.gov

National Women's Health Resource Center
157 Broad Street, Suite 315
Red Bank, NJ 07701
Telephone: (877) 986-9472
Fax: (732) 530-3347
www.healthywomen.org

North American Menopause Society (NAMS)
PO Box 94527
Cleveland, OH 44101
Telephone: (440) 442-7550
www.menopause.org

Pajamas and nightshirts for enduring night sweats:
www.hotcoolwear.com
wjsleepwear.com

PowerSurge, An Online Menopause Community
www.power-surge.com

Women's Health Initiative
National Heart Lung and Blood Institute
NHLBI Health Information Center
Attention: Web Site
P.O. Box 30105
Bethesda, MD 20824-0105
(301) 592-8573
www.nhlbi.nih.gov/whi/

General Health

Centers for Disease Control and Prevention (CDC)
1600 Clifton Road
Atlanta, GA 30333
(800) 311-3435
www.cdc.gov

ivillage.com
www.ivillage.com

Mayo Clinic Health Information
www.mayoclinic.com

National Institute on Aging
National Information Center
PO Box 8057
Gaithersburg, MD 20898
(800) 222-2225
www.nia.nih.gov

National Library of Medicine (Health Information)
National Institutes of Health
Medline Plus
http://medlineplus.gov/

The Alexander Foundation for Women's Health
www.afwh.org

Complementary and Alternative Therapies

Acupuncture Resources for Patients
www.acupuncture.com

American Botanical Council
www.herbalgram.org

American Massage Therapy Association
820 Davis St.
Evanston, IL 60201
www.amtamassage.org

ConsumerLab.com
ConsumerLab.com, LLC
(evaluates quality of herbs, vitamins, dietary and nutritional
   supplements)
333 Mamaroneck Avenue
White Plains, NY 10605
(914) 722-9149
www.consumerlab.com

**National Center for Complementary and Alternative Medicine
(NCCAM)**
PO Box 7923
Gaithersburg, MD 20898
(888) 644-6226
www.nccam.nih.gov

Natural Medicines Comprehensive Database
begun in 1999 and updated daily, this site provides an evaluation
   by 50 clinical pharmacists and physicians for a comprehensive
   listing of brand-name products and their ingredients
www.naturaldatabase.com

Office of Dietary Supplements
National Institutes of Health
Bethesda, MD 20892
http://*dietary-supplements.info.nih.gov/*

Cancer Resources

American Cancer Society
National Home Office
1599 Clifton Road
Atlanta, GA 30329
(800) ACS-2345 or (800) 227-2345
www.cancer.org

Breast Cancer Education Web site:
www.breastcancer.org/

Clinical Trials: A Service of the National Institutes of Health
(linking patients to medical research)
www.clinicaltrials.gov

Susan G. Komen Breast Cancer Foundation
5005 LBJ Freeway, Suite 250
Dallas, TX 75244
Telephone: (972) 855-1600
Helpline: (800) I'M-AWARE
www.komen.org

Wellness Community
919 18th St. NW, Suite 54
Washington, DC 20006
(202) 659-9709
www.wellness-community.org

Caregiver Stress

National Family Caregiver Support Program
(funded through Older Americans Act)
http://www.4woman.gov/faq/caregiver.htm#4

National Eldercare Locator
800-677-1116
www.eldercare.org

National Family Caregivers Association
800-896-3650
www.nfcacares.org

Children of Aging Parents
800-227-7294
www.caps4caregivers.org
www.senioroptions.com
www.natl-eldercare-service.com
www.careguide.net
For nursing homes:
www.achca.org
For legal and financial issues:
National Association of Elder Law Attorneys
520-881-4005
www.naela.org

Professional Geriatric Care Managers
520-881-8008
www.caremanager.org

National Adult Day Services Association
www.ncoa.org

Osteoporosis

NIH Osteoporosis and Related Bone Diseases-National Resource Center
1232 22nd St. NW
Washington, DC 20037
(800) 624-BONE or (800) 624-3663
www.osteo.org

National Osteoporosis Foundation
1232 22nd St. NW
Washington, DC 20037-1292
(202) 223.2226
www.nof.org

Urinary Incontinence

American Urological Association
www.urologyhealth.org

National Association for Continence
PO Box 1019
Charleston, SC 29402
800-BLADDER or (800) 252-3337
www.nafc.org

Simon Foundation (for urinary incontinence)
PO Box 815
Wilmette, IL 60091
800-23SIMON
www.simonfoundation.org

Domestic Violence/Abuse

National Domestic Violence/Abuse Hotline
PO Box 161810
Austin, TX 78716
(800) 799-SAFE or 800-799-7233
(800) 787-3224 (TTY)
If you are being abused, do not go to the Web site below in case
   your computer is monitored. Call the above hotline 24 hours a
   day on a safe phone. They will help you find a local shelter.
   The staff is bilingual, or can direct you to a language line.
www.ndvh.com

Office on Violence Against Women
US Department of Justice
810 7th St. NW
Washington, DC 20531
(202) 307-6026
If you are being abused, do not go to the Web site below in case
   your computer is monitored. Call the National Domestic Vio-
   lence/Abuse hotline (800-799-SAFE) 24 hours a day, using a
   safe phone. They will help you find a local shelter. The staff is
   bilingual, or can direct you to a language line.
www.ojp.usdoj.gov/vawo/

SAFE

Stop Abuse For Everyone
PO Box 951
Tualatin, OR 97062
If you are being abused, do not go to the Web site below in case
   your computer is monitored. Call the National Domestic Vio-
   lence/Abuse hotline 24 hours a day on a safe phone (800-799-
   SAFE). They will help you find a local shelter. The staff is
   bilingual, or can direct you to a language line.
www.safe4all.org

Weight Management

American Obesity Association
1250 24th St. NW, Suite 300
Washington, DC 20037
(202) 776-7711
www.obesity.org

Shape Up America and the 10,000 Steps Program
www.shapeup.org

Active Network
(articles and events for your favorite physical activity)
www.active.com

Center for Nutrition Policy and Promotion
United States Department of Agriculture
www.usda.gov/cnpp
www.nutrition.gov

Division of Nutrition and Physical Activity
National Center for Chronic Disease Prevention
and Health Promotion,
Centers for Disease Control and Prevention
4770 Buford Highway, NE, MS/K-24
Atlanta GA 30341-3717
(770) 488-5820
http://www.cdc.gov/nccdphp/dnpa/

Cardiovascular Disease

American Heart Association
7272 Greenville Avenue
Dallas, TX 75231
800-AHA-USA-1 or (800) 242-8721
www.americanheart.org

American Stroke Association
National Center
7272 Greenville Avenue
Dallas, TX 75231
888-4-STROKE or 888-478-7653
www.strokeassociation.org

Agency for Healthcare Research and Quality
John M. Eisenberg Building
540 Gaither Road
Rockville, MD 20850
(301) 427-1550
www.ahrq.gov/research/womheart

The Heart Truth Campaign
National Heart, Lung, and Blood Institute
Attention: *The Heart Truth*
PO Box 30105
Bethesda, MD 20824-0105
(301) 592-8573, TTY: (240) 629-3255
www.hearttruth.gov

Endocrine Disorders (Diabetes and Thyroid Disease)

American Association of Clinical Endocrinologists
1000 Riverside Ave., Suite 205
Jacksonville, FL 32204
(904) 353-7878
www.aace.com

American Diabetes Association
ATTN: National Call Center
1701 North Beauregard Street
Alexandria, VA 22311
800-DIABETES or 800-342-2383
www.diabetes.org

Mental Health, Depression, and Social Isolation

Girlfriends for Life
www.girlfriendsforlife.org

National Institute of Mental Health (NIMH)
Office of Communications
6001 Executive Boulevard, Room 8184, MSC 9663
Bethesda, MD 20892-9663
(866) 615-6464
www.nimh.nih.gov

The Red Hat Society
Fun and Friendship After Age 50
www.redhatsociety.com

Sexual Dysfunction

Institute of Sexual Medicine
Boston University
715 Albany St.
Boston, MA 02118
(617) 638-8576
www.bumc.bu.edu/sexualmedicine/clinic

Dry Eye and Eye Disorders

Prevent Blindness America
(for information on dry eye and eye screening)
500 East Remington Road
Schaumburg, IL 60173
(800) 331-2020
www.preventblindness.org

Compounding Pharmacies

Women's International Pharmacy
(800) 279-5708
www.womensinternational.com

Directory of Compounding Pharmacies:
http://dmoz.org/Health/Pharmacy/Pharmacies/Compounding/

Sleep

National Heart, Lung, and Blood Institute
Sleep Disorders Research
www.nhlbi.nih.gov/health/prof/sleep/

Sleep Foundation
www.sleepfoundation.org

Appendix A

Appendix B

Hormone Therapies for the Treatment of Menopausal Symptoms

Hormone, How Taken	Product Name (Manufacturer), How Supplied	Type of Hormone	Comments
*Estrogens, By Mouth	Biestrogen [Bi-Est] (compounding pharmacies), Capsules	Micronized estradiol (20%) Micronized estriol (80%)	• Bio-identical estradiol and estriol • Long-term effects of bio-identical hormones unknown • Hormones extracted from wild yam and soy • Tell compounding pharmacy if you have peanut allergy
	Cenestin (Duramed), Tablets	Conjugated estrogens	• Synthetic form of estrogen derived from plant sources
	Estrace (Warner Chilcott), Tablets	Micronized estradiol	• Bio-identical estradiol • Sometimes placed under the tongue
	Estratab (Solvay), Tablets	Esterified estrogens	• Take with milk/food to reduce stomach upset
	Menest (Monarch), Tablets	Esterified estrogens	• Synthesized in the laboratory • Also used for palliative treatment in breast cancer
	Ogen (Pharmacia), Tablets	Estropipate	• Synthesized in laboratory • Recommended for cyclic regimens
	Ortho-Est (Women First), Tablets	Estropipate	• Synthesized in laboratory • Recommended for cyclic regimens

Hormone, How Taken	Product Name (Manufacturer), How Supplied	Type of Hormone	Comments
*Estrogens, By Mouth	Premarin (Wyeth), Tablets	Conjugated Equine Estrogen (CEE)	• Available in many dosages • Most widely studied estrogen • Made from estrogens found in pregnant mare's urine
	Triestrogen [Tri-Est] (compounding pharmacies), Capsules	Micronized estrone (10%) Micronized estradiol (10%) Micronized estriol (80%)	• Bio-identical estrone, estradiol, and estriol • Long-term effects of bio-identical hormones unknown • Hormones extracted from wild yam and soy • Tell compounding pharmacy if you have peanut allergy
	Activella (Novo Nordisk), Tablets	Estradiol + norethindrone acetate	• Bio-identical estradiol • One combined tablet taken daily
	Biestrogen with progesterone (compounding pharmacies), Capsules	Micronized estradiol, estriol and micronized progesterone	• Bio-identical hormones • Can be compounded in various strengths and percentages • Tell compounding pharmacy if you have peanut allergy
	FemHRT (Warner Chilcott), Tablets	ethinyl estradiol + norethindrone acetate	• Tablets taken continuously

Hormone, How Taken	Product Name (Manufacturer), How Supplied	Type of Hormone	Comments
*Estrogens, By Mouth	Prefest (Monarch), Tablets	Estradiol and norgestimate	• Estrogen made from soy • Taken daily in sequence: 3 tablets of estradiol, then 3 tablets of estradiol and norgestimate, then repeat
	Premphase (Wyeth), Tablets	Conjugated equine estrogen (14 tablets), then conjugated equine estrogen plus medroxyprogesterone acetate (MPA) (14 tablets)	• One tablet per day taken in sequence starting with estrogen followed by estrogen plus progestin • You will get a period when you stop the sequence of pills containing progestin
	Prempro (Wyeth), Tablets	Conjugated equine estrogen and medroxyprogesterone acetate (MPA)	• Available in many dosages • Contains the most widely studied estrogen • Manufactured from estrogens found in pregnant mare's urine • One tablet taken daily
	Triestrogen with progesterone (compounding pharmacies), Capsules	Micronized estradiol, estriol, and estrone and micronized progesterone	• Bio-identical hormones • Can be compounded in various doses and percentages • Tell compounding pharmacy if you have peanut allergy

Hormone, How Taken	Product Name (Manufacturer), How Supplied	Type of Hormone	Comments
*Estrogens, Applied to Skin	Alora (Watson), Patch	Estradiol	• Bio-identical estradiol • Patch may be cut smaller for smaller dosage • Patch is changed twice a week
	Climara (Berlex), Patch	Estradiol	• Bio-identical estradiol • Patch may be cut smaller to make smaller dosage • Patch changed once a week
	Esclim (Women First), Patch	Estradiol	• Bio-identical estradiol • Do not cut this patch • Change patch twice a week • Do not apply patch to breast
	Estraderm (Novartis), Patch	Estradiol	• Bio-identical estradiol • Change patch twice a week • Do not cut this patch • Do not apply patch to breast
	EstroGel (Solvay), Gel	Estradiol	• Bio-identical estradiol • Gel applied once daily to arm, from shoulder to wrists, like a skin cream • Takes several minutes to dry • Odorless • Measured doses from a non-aerosol pump

Hormone, How Taken	Product Name (Manufacturer), How Supplied	Type of Hormone	Comments
*Estrogens, Applied to Skin	Estrosorb (Novavax), Cream	Estradiol emulsion	• Bio-identical estradiol • Cream rubbed into thigh • Takes several minutes to dry • Supplied in packets • Be sure it is fully dry prior to dressing
	Vivelle-Dot (Novogyne), Patch	Estradiol	• Smallest available patch to treat menopausal symptoms • Changed twice a week • Do not apply patch to breast
*Combination Estrogen + Progestin, Applied to the Skin	Climara Pro (Berlex), Patch	Estradiol + levonorgestrel	• Patch applied once weekly • Apply to clean, dry skin of lower abdomen • Rotate sites, avoid waistline • Never put patch on breasts • Bio-identical estradiol
	CombiPatch (Novogyne), Patch	Estradiol + norethindrone acetate	• Both hormones in one patch • Bio-identical estradiol • Progestin is synthetic • Comes in two strengths/sizes of patch • Change patches every 3 to 4 days • Use on dry, clean skin

Appendix B

Hormone, How Taken	Product Name (Manufacturer), How Supplied	Type of Hormone	Comments
Progestogen Only Products	Amen (Carnrick), Cycrin (Wyeth-Ayerst), Tablets	Medroxyprogesterone acetate (MPA)	• Range of dosages available • Often used to treat abnormal uterine bleeding of perimenopause
	Aygestin (Barr), Tablets	Norethindrone acetate	• Often used to treat abnormal uterine bleeding • Sometimes has fewer side effects than MPA
	Megace (Bristol Myers Squibb), Tablets	Megesterol acetate	• Also used as a treatment for advanced cancer of the breast • May be effective treatment of hot flashes in women with breast cancer • Can cause intestinal disturbance, weight gain, chest pain, edema, high blood pressure, high glucose levels, rash, fever, insomnia, urinary frequency, weakness, decreased sex drive, indigestion
	Mirena (Berlex), IUD (Intrauterine device)	Levonorgestrel	• Primary use is birth control, but may be sufficient progesterone to protect against overgrowth of the uterine lining

Hormone, How Taken	Product Name (Manufacturer), How Supplied	Type of Hormone	Comments
Progestogen Only Products	Pro-Gest (Transitions for Health), Cream	Progesterone	• Bio-identical progesterone • Available without prescription or by prescription from compounding pharmacies
	Prometrium (Solvay), Capsules	Micronized progesterone with peanut oil	• Bioidentical progesterone • Do not take if you have a peanut allergy
	Provera (Pharmacia), Tablets	Medroxyprogesterone acetate (MPA)	• Most studied progestin • Often used to treat abnormal uterine bleeding • Range of dosages available
*Combination Estrogen + Testosterone, By Mouth	Estratest HS (Solvay) and Estratest (Solvay), Syntest (Syntho) and Menogen (Breckinridge), Tablets	Esterified estrogens + methytestosterone	• FDA-approved for treatment of hot flashes when other hormone treatments have not provided relief • Although not FDA-approved for improving libido, this combination may be prescribed to help both hot flashes and low libido
*Estrogen + Testosterone, Combination Injection	Depo-Testadiol (Pfizer), Depotestogen (Hyrex), Injection	Estradiol cyprionate and testosterone cyprionate	• Given monthly • FDA-approved for treatment of hot flashes when other hormone treatments have not provided relief

Hormone, How Taken	Product Name (Manufacturer), How Supplied	Type of Hormone	Comments
*Estrogen + Testosterone, Combination Injection	Depo-Testadiol (Pfizer), Depotestogen (Hyrex), Injection (continued)	Estradiol cyprionate and testosterone cyprionate	• Although not FDA-approved for improving libido, this combination may be prescribed to help both hot flashes and low libido
*Estrogens, Progesterone, Testosterone for Vaginal/ Genital Use	Crinone (Serono), Vaginal Gel	Progesterone	• Bio-identical to human progesterone • Prefilled applicator • This gel is usually prescribed for women with infertility to enhance the possibility of implantation
	Estrace (Warner Chilcott), Vaginal Cream	Micronized 17-beta-estradiol	• Bio-identical estradiol • Usually prescribed daily, then 1 to 3 times per week as needed • Often prescribed when waiting for other prescribed estrogens to take effect on vaginal dryness
	Estring (Pharmacia), Vaginal Ring	Micronized 17-beta-estradiol	• Bio-identical estradiol • Replaced once every 3 months • Relieves vaginal symptoms • Progestin may not be needed • May provide support for urinary incontinence

Appendix B

Hormone, How Taken	Product Name (Manufacturer), How Supplied	Type of Hormone	Comments
*Estrogens, Progesterone, Testosterone for Vaginal/Genital Use	Femring (Warner Chilcott), Vaginal Ring	Estradiol acetate	• If you can feel it inside, it is not positioned correctly • Replaced once every 3 months • Relieves systemic and vaginal symptoms • May provide support for urinary incontinence
	Ogen (Pharmacia Upjohn), Vaginal Cream	Estropipate	• Contains some but not all bio-identical estrogen
	Premarin (Wyeth), Vaginal Cream	Conjugated equine estrogen	• Estrogen manufactured from urine of pregnant mares • Can be used with or without an applicator
	First Testosterone (Cutis Pharma), Cream or Ointment	Testosterone proprionate	• Synthesized testosterone from plants • Some women report improvement in libido and sexual function • Applied to the clitoris and vulvo-vaginal area

Appendix B

Hormone, How Taken	Product Name (Manufacturer), How Supplied	Type of Hormone	Comments
*Estrogens, Progesterone, Testosterone for Vaginal/Genital Use	Vagifem (Novo Nordisk), Vaginal Tablets	Estradiol hemihydrate	• Preloaded tablets in disposable applicator • Insert once daily for 2 weeks, then twice weekly

*If you still have a uterus and are taking oral estrogen or some estrogens applied to the skin or vagina, a progestin is needed to protect your uterus lining from over-growth.

281

Glossary

Acupuncture: A form of alternative medicine that uses tiny needles inserted along qi (energy) lines (meridians).

Adipose tissue: Fat tissue. Androgens are changed to estrogen (estrone) in the adipose tissue.

Adrenal glands: The two small endocrine glands located just above the kidneys. The adrenal glands secrete sex hormones, cortisol, and epinephrine.

Aerobic exercise: Exercise intended to strengthen your heart, such as running, cycling, or brisk walking by increasing your breathing and heart rate, this type of exercise helps your body burn off fat, and helps control cholesterol.

Alternative therapies: Therapies or practices used in place of conventional medical treatments.

Alzheimer's disease: Degenerative brain disorder that gradually causes disorientation, confusion, and memory loss.

Amenorrhea: Absence of menstruation for 3 months or more.

Androgen: Although much more common in men, these hormones are also present in women. Androgens are secreted by the ovary and the adrenal gland. Androgens, such as testosterone and DHEA, are converted in fat tissue to one form of estrogen (estrone). They are important for libido, and balance with estrogen for sexual development.

Andropause: Short for androgenpause. Applied to men, it's a period of time that is speculated to be similar to menopause in women; a time of shifting hormones and midlife changes.

Anorexia nervosa: A disorder characterized by fear of becoming obese, thinking the body is larger than it really is, severe weight loss, and an aversion to food. Once thought to only affect teenage girls, it is now recognized in women of all ages.

Anterior pituitary gland: The part of the pituitary gland, which is situated at the base of the brain, that releases follicle stimulating hormone (FSH) and luteinizing hormone (LH) as part of the menstrual cycle.

Antihistamine: A medication intended to reduce allergic reactions, also dries mucous membranes like the mouth and vagina.

Antioxidant: Substance that helps reduce damage that can cause cancer or accelerate the aging process. Antioxidants include Vitamins C and E, betacarotene, flavonoids, and lycopene.

Binge eating disorder: A disorder characterized by eating very large quantities of food in short periods of time, usually leads to being overweight or obese.

Bio-identical hormone: Hormones manufactured in a laboratory from wild yam or soy that have the exact same chemical makeup as the hormones made in the body. Sometimes called "natural" hormones.

Biopsy: A piece of tissue removed from the body and examined for abnormalities.

Black cohosh: An herb in the buttercup family used frequently in Native American medicine for a variety of ailments, including rheumatism, colds, constipation, backache and gynecological disorders. Also called black snakeroot, bugwort, bugbane, rattleroot, rattletop, macrotys, and squawroot. Used by many women to treat hot flashes.

Body Mass Index (BMI): A measurement of body size that includes both height and weight. It is calculated by dividing your weight (in pounds) by your height (in inches) squared, multiplied by 704.5.

Botanical: Any plant, although used mostly in reference to herbs or flowers, that is used medicinally.

Bulimia: An eating disorder that usually includes episodes of binge eating (eating very large amounts of food) and purging (forcing vomiting or diarrhea to get food out of the system).

Cardiovascular: Relating to the heart or blood vessels.

Cataract: A cloudy lens of the eye that leads to vision problems and if untreated, can lead to blindness. Is usually surgically corrected.

Chlamydia: A common bacterial infection transmitted vaginally, orally, or anally during sex that may have no symptoms. It can cause burning and inflammation of the urethra, and vaginal discharge. It can lead to infertility if untreated.

Chloasma: Patches of darkened skin that may result from aging, sun, or as a medication side effect.

Chronic obstructive pulmonary disease (COPD): A chronic lung disease that causes slowed or difficult breathing, wheezing, and increased mucous.

Clitoris: Female counterpart of the penis that becomes erect with sexual stimulation. Unlike the penis, the clitoris does not house the urethra. The clitoris is located just in front of the urethral opening under a "hood" of tissue, and is sensitive to stimulation.

Cognition: Mental processes that are related to knowledge gathering, judgment, reasoning, imagining, and memory.

Cognitive: Pertaining to the areas of the brain that control reasoning, judgment, knowing, imagining, and memory.

Complementary therapies: Therapies or practices used with conventional medical treatments.

Compounding pharmacy: A pharmacy that specializes in preparing medications (oral, suppositories, creams, tinctures, etc.) that are put together in specific percentages by the compounding pharmacist as prescribed by a clinician. Many compounding pharmacies also carry brand name medications, as well.

Conjugated estrogens: A blend of several manufactured estrogens in one product used in HT.

Conjugated equine estrogen (CEE): The most common form of estrogen used in hormone therapy (HT); a blend of estrogens extracted from the urine of pregnant mares.

Continuous combined regimen: A method of taking hormone therapy (HT) in which the woman takes estrogen and progestin every day without stopping.

Coping skills training: Learning new ways to solve problems usefully

by learning how to analyze a problem, identify possible solutions, decide how to reach the solution, and make it happen.

Corpus luteum: Formed in the ovary as a result of the release of the mature egg. It becomes a yellowish color and secretes progesterone.

Cyclic regimen: A method of taking hormone therapy (HT) in which the woman takes an estrogen tablet once a day for 25 days of the month. For the last 10 to 14 days of estrogen, she adds a progestin tablet, and takes both estrogen and progestin pills each day until day 25 of the month. She takes nothing from day 26 to the end of the month.

Dementia: Condition marked by memory loss, lack of ability to attend to personal care, personality changes, impaired reasoning, and bouts of disorientation.

DHEA (dehydroepiandrosterone): A steroid that has androgen effects.

Dietary supplement: Any substance that is added to the diet, such as vitamins, minerals, or herbs, in addition to what your body already takes in. Some progesterone creams are also termed dietary supplements even though you don't eat them.

Diuretic: Substance or medication that causes an increase in urine excretion. Caffeine is an example of a naturally occurring mild diuretic.

Douching (vaginal): The act of using water mixed with medication or cleansing agent with the intent of hygiene or treatment of the vagina.

Dyspareunia: Pain with sexual intercourse.

Elemental calcium: The calcium that your body absorbs and uses.

Endometrial cancer: Cancer of the lining of the uterus.

Endometrial hyperplasia: An abnormal thickening or overgrowth of the lining of the uterus. This may lead to cancer.

Endometrial lining: The lining of the uterus that is shed during menstruation. If allowed to thicken without shedding, endometrial hyperplasia or endometrial cancer may develop.

Endometriosis: A painful condition characterized by the abnormal presence of endometrial tissue outside the uterus, such as on an ovary, the colon, or bladder.

Endometrium: The inner layer of the uterus. The lining of the endometrium is shed during menstruation.

Endorphins: Brain chemicals responsible for reducing pain and affecting emotions.

Episiotomy: Incision made in the perineum to ease delivery of a baby.

Erectile dysfunction: Inability to make the penis rigid.

Esterified estrogens Estropipates, Ethinyl estradiol: Manufactured forms of estrogen used in hormone therapy (HT).

Estradiol: The most potent of the naturally occurring estrogens in the human body and the main estrogen of the reproductive years. Also called E2.

Estriol: Estriol (E3) is the main estrogen of pregnancy and is secreted by the placenta. It is also present in women who are not pregnant as a byproduct of E1 and E2.

Estrogen: Known as a female sex hormone although it is also found in men in small amounts. It is primarily secreted by the ovary in response to follicle stimulating hormone (FSH). Estrogens used in hormone therapy (HT) can be manufactured using certain plants, or from pregnant mare's urine.

Estrogen progestin therapy (EPT): Estrogen- and progestin-containing products that are used in combination for the treatment of menopausal symptoms.

Estrogen receptors: Sites in the human body where estrogen binds and affects cell functions. Estrogen receptors can be found in parts of the brain, the eyes, heart, lungs, breasts, liver, colon, reproductive organs, urinary system, blood vessels, and bone.

Estrogen therapy (ET): Estrogen-containing products that are used in the treatment of perimenopausal and menopausal symptoms. Estrogen taken by itself for the treatment of menopausal symptoms.

Estrone: The main estrogen of the postmenopausal phase, and is also present in small amounts in men and children. Also called E1.

Extract: A concentrated form of a substance, e.g., an herb.

Fallopian tubes: The slim straw-like tubes that lead from the ovaries to the top of either side of the uterus. The egg travels from the ovary through the fallopian tube to the uterus.

Female sexual dysfunction (FSD): A medical condition characterized by symptoms including lack of desire for sex, lack of arousal during sex, lack of ability to reach orgasm, or pain during intercourse.

Fibroid: A type of non-cancerous tumor, also called leiomyomas, found in the uterus.

Final menstrual period (FMP): The last menstrual period before menopause. Like menopause, the FMP can only be identified in hindsight.

Follicle: A sac of immature "eggs" in the ovary stimulated to grow by the follicle stimulating hormone (FSH) and estrogen. When estrogen levels get high enough, luteinizing hormone (LH) is released too so that the dominant follicle expels a mature egg from the ovary.

Follicle stimulating hormone (FSH): A hormone released from the anterior pituitary gland to stimulate the growth of follicles in the ovary. Estrogen levels also rise in response to FSH.

Glucosamine condroitin: A supplement that can help joint pain and arthritis. It provides nutrition to the cartilage around the joints.

Gonadotropin-releasing hormone (GnRH): A hormone that is released from the hypothalamus to stimulate production of luteinizing hormone (LH) and follicle stimulating hormone (FSH).

Guided imagery: A process used to help someone imagine a picture or a place. It is used during psychotherapy as a way to focus on problems, or during uncomfortable procedures like chemotherapy to divert attention away from pain and nausea. It is also commonly used to assist with relaxation (e.g., imagining a gentle stream with ducks floating on it).

Hippocampus: A part of the brain that helps with memory.

Homocysteine: An amino acid that is being studied for its role in increasing heart disease and osteoporosis. Vitamin B and folate are known to reduce homocysteine levels.

Hormone therapy (HT): An umbrella term that describes the use of estrogen, progesterone, or some combination of the two, and sometimes testosterone, to treat the symptoms of menopause.

Hot flashes: Sensations of heat that often begin at the head and spread over the entire body. The hot flash accompanies perimenopause and postmenopause for many women. It occurs with an increase in lutenizing hormone, does not provide a health hazard, may be accompanied by sweating, and can cause significant discomfort or awaken women from sleep.

HPO axis (hypothalamus-pituitary-ovarian axis): The feedback system that regulates levels of estrogen, progesterone, follicle stimulating hormone (FSH), gonadotropin releasing hormone (GnRH), and luteinizing hormone.

Human papilloma virus (HPV): A virus that is transmitted sexually. Some types of HPV are associated with cancer of the cervix.

Hyperthyroidism: Overproduction of thyroid hormone.

Hysterectomy: Removal of the uterus.

Idiopathic: Having no known cause.

Idiopathic ovarian insufficiency: The loss of ovarian function (and therefore fertility) in a woman under the age of 40, resulting in menopause. It is usually associated with other health conditions, and can sometimes be temporary.

Inactive ingredient: A filler or sometimes a preservative used in the making of some medications and supplements. Although not intended to have any effect on the body, inactive ingredients can sometimes cause reactions.

Incontinence (urinary): Inability to hold urine.

Induced menopause: Permanent menopause that is not natural; can happen as a result of removal of the ovaries, chemotherapy, or radiation to the pelvis.

Injectable: Given into the muscle or fat tissue using a needle with a syringe attached.

Insulin resistance: Insulin has difficulty carrying sugar into body cells (the cells are resistant). High levels of insulin, and sometimes blood sugar, result. People with insulin resistance are at higher risk for developing diabetes.

Iron deficiency anemia: Blood disorder characterized by loss of oxygen-carrying blood cells either by inadequate iron intake or by loss of blood.

Irregular periods: Shorter, longer, lighter, or heavier than the usual period.

Isoflavones: A type of phytoestrogen found most notably in soy and red clover.

Kegel exercises: Tensing and releasing muscles that surround the urethra and vagina. Kegels are intended to help relieve stress incontinence, and also to strengthen vaginal and pelvic muscles.

Lactation: The period of time when the mammary glands in the breasts produce milk.

L-arginine: A substance known to increase blood flow to the clitoris.

Libido: Sex drive.

Lipids: Generally considered to be the fats and cholesterol found in blood. Higher density lipids are the "good" fats, and the lower density lipids are the "bad" fats.

Lubrication (vaginal): Using a water-soluble substance to make sexual intercourse more comfortable if normal vaginal lubrication isn't possible either because of lack of arousal or because of vaginal atrophy.

Lutein: The yellowish pigment that gives the corpus luteum its yellowish color.

Luteinizing hormone (LH): A hormone released from the pituitary gland that stimulates ovulation during the menstrual cycle. It also has a role in causing hot flashes.

Macular degeneration: The most common cause of blindness in postmenopausal women. Caused by a deterioration in part of the retina, resulting in a progressive loss of central vision.

Mediterranean diet: A diet high in whole grains, vegetables, tomatoes, olive oil, and moderate amounts of red wine.

Melasma: Patches of darkened skin that occur as a result of exposure to sun, aging, or as a side effect of medication.

Melatonin: A pineal gland hormone important for the sleep-wake cycle and used to treat jet lag or sleep disturbances in shift workers, but has not been proven to improve sleep onset or decrease night waking.

Menarche: The first menstrual period.

Menopause: Specific point in time occurring after 12 consecutive months without a menstrual period that does not have another identifiable cause such as illness or medication.

Menopause transition: The time period before and up to the final menstrual period when hormonal changes occur.

Menstrual life: The number of menstrual periods in your lifetime.

Menstrual period: The blood flow that occurs approximately every 28 to 30 days in a reproductive-aged woman when the top layer of the lining of the internal uterus wall sheds.

Menstruation: The process of discharging the blood and endometrial debris during the menstrual period.

Micronized: When a product is prepared with very small particle sizes, as opposed to fewer larger particles, so it has a larger surface area and is better absorbed in the intestines.

Migraine: A headache, usually on one side of the head, which causes severe pain and is sometimes accompanied by nausea, vomiting, and vision disturbances.

Mind-body interventions: Any therapy or process engaged in to use the mind as a healing tool for the body.

Monosodium glutamate: A chemical substance used for seasoning food.

Monounsaturated fats: Fats derived from plants that are considered healthier than saturated fats from animal sources. Olive oil and safflower oil are examples.

Oophorectomy: Removal of one ovary. Bilateral oophorectomy is removal of both ovaries.

Osteoarthritis: Inflammation and stiffness of the joints that usually occurs in older people as a result of deterioration of the cartilage around the joints.

Osteoporosis: A reduction in bone density that makes bone more fragile and susceptible to fractures.

Over-the-counter (OTC): Describes medications, herbs, or supplements that can be bought without a prescription.

Ovulation: The release of an egg (ovum) from the ovary stimulated by luteinizing hormone. It usually occurs approximately 14 days before the first day of the menstrual period. It is sometimes accompanied by mild to moderate pain called "mittelschmertz" (pain at the middle of the menstrual cycle that accompanies ovulation).

Paced breathing: A method of breathing used for relaxation. Breathe in for 4 counts, hold for 7 counts, breathe out for 8 counts.

Palpitations: Abnormally fast or irregular heartbeats.

Panic attack: Sudden onset of intense apprehension, fear, or impending doom accompanied by physical symptoms such as nausea, sweating, and heart palpitations.

Parkinson's disease: A brain disorder characterized by abnormal movements, tremors, weakness, and sometimes paralysis. Usually affects people 50 years of age or older.

Perimenopause: Time period before and up to menopause, including the 12 months of no menses when symptoms of hormonal changes occur; can last up to 8 to 10 years.

Pessary: A device that's fitted into the vagina and provides some support between the urethra and the vaginal wall. It is fitted by a urologist or gynecologist, but may be removed, cleaned, and inserted again at home.

Physiologic: Pertaining to body function.

Phytoestrogens: Weak estrogen-like substances that are in plants. Can be eaten in whole foods, such as soy, or extracted from red clover in the form of isoflavones and made into supplements.

Placebo: An inactive substance that contains no medication or active ingredient to be given to participants in a clinical trial to determine the effectiveness of a particular medication or substance.

Positive and negative feedback systems: Certain hormones or substances are released in response to either high or low levels of another hormone or substance.

Postmenopausal: Pertaining to the time period following menopause.

Premature or early menopause: Permanent natural menopause occurring in a woman who is younger than 40 years of age.

Premature ovarian failure: The loss of ovarian function (and therefore fertility) in a woman under the age of 40, resulting in menopause. It is usually associated with other health conditions, and can sometimes be temporary.

Prescription: An instruction from a licensed clinician like a physician, a nurse practitioner, a midwife, or a physician's assistant that provides for a medication or device to be issued by a pharmacy.

Progesterone: A female sex hormone that is responsible for the changes in the uterus, especially during the part of the menstrual cycle that is preparing the uterine lining for a fertilized egg, and that helps to sustain pregnancy. It is also the female hormone that protects the endometrial lining of the uterus from thickening too much in response to estrogen.

Progesterone receptor sites: Sites in the human body where progesterone binds and affects cell functions. Progesterone receptors can be found in parts of the brain, heart, lungs, breasts, pancreas, reproductive organs, blood vessels, and bone.

Progestin therapy (PT): Progestin taken by itself for the treatment of menopausal symptoms.

Progestins: Any manufactured progesterone. They can be used to prevent overgrowth of the uterine lining to prevent the risk for endometrial cancer, stabilize the uterine lining during irregular bleeding, help manage menopause symptoms, and to sustain pregnancy.

Progestogens: Refers to either progesterone made in the body or to progestins manufactured for the purposes of hormone therapy.

Progressive relaxation: A way to relax by tensing and releasing muscles one at a time.

Puberty: Stage of adolescence at which a male or female becomes capable of reproduction.

Pulsed regimen: A method of taking hormone therapy (HT) in which estrogen is taken for 3 days, and then progestin is added to the estrogen for 3 days, then estrogen alone for 3 days, and then estrogen with progestin for 3 days, and so on, in a repeated fashion.

Resistive exercises: Exercises where the muscles must push and pull against force, such as weight training and swimming.

Retinoids: A form of Vitamin A found in beef, eggs, shrimp, fish, milk, and certain kinds of cheeses.

Rheumatoid arthritis: A form of joint inflammation and stiffness that affects women more than men, and usually starts at an earlier age than osteoarthritis. The joints can later become deformed and cause considerable disability. Rheumatoid arthritis is also an autoimmune disorder, and can be diagnosed by examining the blood for a particular factor.

Salpingo-oophorectomy: Removal of fallopian tubes and ovaries.

Sedative: A medication intended to produce a calming effect.

Sequential cyclic regimen: A method of taking hormone therapy (HT) in which the woman takes estrogen every day continuously, and adds a progestin on days 1 through 14, or days 14 through 28. She has a period after she finishes taking the progestin every month.

Serotonin: A brain substance associated with good mood and sleep. Some antidepressants (selective serotonin reuptake inhibitors) aid in increasing levels of serotonin.

17-beta estradiol: The most commonly used bio-identical manufactured estrogen.

Sexually transmitted infections (STIs): Formerly called sexually transmitted diseases. Infections contracted during sexual contact, such as herpes, gonorrhea, syphilis, human immunodeficiency virus (HIV), several forms of hepatitis including B and C, trichomoniasis, and chlamydia.

Sleep hygiene: A group of healthy practices that contribute to a good night's sleep.

Soy: The substance derived from soybeans, a protein-rich, low-fat legume.

Spermicide: A jelly-type or foam substance used with condoms and diaphragms to kill sperm as a form of birth control. Some types of spermicide also reduce the risk for some sexually transmitted infections.

Stem cells: Unspecialized cells that eventually develop into specialized cells, such as those found in the ovary.

Stressor: Anything that causes stress.

Sublingual: Under the tongue.

Tai chi: A form of exercise that combines meditation and flexibility training.

Tamoxifen: A medication often given to patients with estrogen-linked breast cancer to help prevent recurrence.

Temporary menopause: Temporary loss of periods for over 1 year. Occurs when normal function of the ovary is interrupted either by medications, cancer treatments, stress, over exercising, severe weight loss, or for unknown reasons.

Testosterone: A steroid hormone formed by the testes in males, and to a far lesser degree, by the ovary and adrenal glands in women. It is responsible for male characteristics such as a deep voice and facial hair, and is important for normal sexual development and function in women.

Tincture: An alcohol-based liquid preparation used for some herbs.

Topically: Applied to the skin.

Total hysterectomy: Although technically only refers to removal of the uterus, "total" is sometimes used to refer to removal of the uterus, ovaries, and fallopian tubes.

Toxic shock syndrome: A condition characterized by sudden onset of high fever, vomiting, rash, and eventually shock, usually as a result of a blood infection caused by a tampon that has stayed in the vagina too long.

Trichomoniasis: Vaginal inflammation caused by an organism called *Trichomonas vaginalis.* It is usually transmitted during sex.

Triggers: Foods, substances, or activities that prompt a certain response in the body.

TVT surgery: Stands for trans-vaginal-tuck, a surgical procedure in which some tissue is made into a sling-type arrangement that supports the bladder and urethra in the treatment of stress incontinence.

Ultrasound: Use of high frequency sound waves to visualize organs of the body.

Urogenital: Relating to the urinary and the reproductive systems, especially the vagina in women (synonymous with genitourinary).

Uterine prolapse: When the uterus sits at a lower place in the abdominal cavity, or slips into the vagina.

Vaginal atrophy: Shrinkage of the surface layer of cells in the vagina during postmenopause, accompanied by dryness and lack of elasticity of the vagina.

Vaginal discharge: Substance that comes out of the vagina that results from normal mucous production, infection, hormones, overgrowth of normal vaginal bacteria, allergies, irritations, menstrual blood flow, or cancer.

Vaginitis: Inflammation of the vagina.

Vasectomy: The surgery that cuts the vas deferens, the connection from the testis to the urethra in a male, so that sperm cannot be part of the ejaculate.

Vasomotor: The part of the brain that regulates dilation and constriction of blood vessels.

Vasomotor symptoms: Symptoms resulting from irregular function of the part of the brain that controls body heat, usually experienced as hot flashes and sweats that may or may not be followed by feeling cold or chilled.

Wild yam: An herb that was originally used to manufacture progesterone starting in the 1940s. It does not contain progesterone, but instead contains a molecule that is used to manufacture progesterone in a laboratory.

Withdrawal bleeding: Vaginal (period-like) bleeding that occurs after stopping progestin. This bleeding allows the lining of the uterus to shed.

Yoga: A group of breathing exercises and movements intended to improve flexibility and strength, and bring about tranquility.

In addition to the resources listed in Appendix A, the following books and scientific sources were used as references in the preparation of this book.

Alexander I. M., Ruff C., Rousseau M. E., et al. Experiences and perceptions of menopause and midlife health among black women. Paper presented at: Eastern Nursing Research Society (ENRS) 16th Annual Scientific Sessions, Partnerships: Advancing the Research Agenda for Quality Care; April 1–3, 2004, 2004; Quincy, MA.

Alexander I. M., Ruff C., Rousseau M. E., et al. Menopause symptoms and management strategies identified by black women (abstract). *Menop.* 2003;10(6):601.

Alexander I. M., Ruff C. C., Udemezue C. Correlation between lifestyle behaviors and severity of menopausal symptoms in black women; u.d.

Anderson G. L., Limacher M., Assaf A. R., et al. Effects of conjugated equine estrogen in postmenopausal women with hysterectomy: the Women's Health Initiative randomized controlled trial. *JAMA.* 291(14):1701–1712.

Anonymous. eHippocrates. Accessed updated daily, 2004.

Antonijevic I. A., Stalla G. K., Steiger A. Modulation of the sleep electroencephalogram by estrogen replacement in postmenopausal women. *Am J of Obstet Gynec.* 2000;182(2):277–282.

Arlt W., Callies F., Allolio B. DHEA replacement in women with adrenal insufficiency—pharmacokinetics, bioconversion and clinical effects on well-being, sexuality and cognition. *Endoc Res.* 2000;26(4):505–511.

Aslaksen K., Frankendal B.. Effect of oral medroxyprogesterone acetate on menopausal symptoms in patients with endometrial carcinoma. *Acta Obstet Gynec Scand.* 1982;61(5):423–428.

Atkinson C., Compston J. E., Day N. E., Dowsett M., Bingham S. A. The effects of phytoestrogen isoflavones on bone density in women: a double-blind, randomized, placebo-controlled trial. *Am J Clin Nutr.* 2004;79(2):326–333.

Atkinson C., Warren R. M., Sala E., et al. Red-clover-derived isoflavones and mammographic breast density: a double-blind, randomized, placebo-controlled trial. *Breast Cancer Res.* 2004;6(3):R170–R179.

Ayas N. T., White D. P., Manson J. E., et al. A prospective study of sleep duration and coronary heart disease in women. *Arch Int Med.* 2003;163(2):205–209.

Bachman G. A., Leiblum S. R. The impact of hormones on menopausal sexuality: A literature review. *Menop.* 2004;11(1):120–130.

Barton D., Loprinzi C., Quella S., Sloan J., Pruthi S., Novotny P. Depomedroxyprogesterone acetate for hot flashes. *J Pain Symp Manag.* 2002;24(6):603–607.

Barton D. L., Loprinzi C. L., Quella S. K., et al. Prospective evaluation of Vitamin E for hot flashes in breast cancer survivors. *J Clin Oncol.* 1998;16(2):495–500.

Bastian L. A., Smith C. M., Nanda K. Is this woman perimenopausal? *JAMA.* 2003;289(7):895–902.

Berman J. R., Berman L. A., Werbin T. J., Flaherty E. E., Leahy N. M., Goldstein I. Clinical evaluation of female sexual function: effects of age and estrogen status on subjective and physiologic sexual responses. *Int J Impot Res.* 2001;11(Suppl 1):S31–S38.

Bertelli G., Venturini M., Del Mastro L., et al. Intramuscular depot medroxyprogesterone versus oral megestrol for the control of postmenopausal hot flashes in breast cancer patients: a randomized study. *Ann Oncol.* 2002;13(6):883–888.

Blumel J. E., Castelo-Branco C., Binfa L., et al. Quality of life after the menopause: a population study. *Maturitas.* 2000;34(1):17–23.

Boothby L. A., Doering P. L., Kipersztok S. K. Biodentical hormone therapy: A review. *Menop.* 2004;11(3):356–367.

Brincat M., Versi E., Moniz C. F., Magos A., de Trafford J., Studd J. W. Skin collagen changes in postmenopausal women receiving different regimens of estrogen therapy. *Obstet Gynecol.* 1987;70(1):123–127.

Brincat M., Versi E., O'Dowd T., et al. Skin collagen changes in postmenopausal women receiving oestradiol gel. *Maturitas.* 1987;9(1):1–5.

Brincat M., Yuen A. W., Studd J. W., Montgomery J., Magos A. L., Savvas M. Response of skin thickness and metacarpal index to estradiol therapy in postmenopausal women. *Obstet Gyneco.* 1987;70(4):538–541.

Bromberger J. T., Matthews K. A., Kuller L. H., Wing R. R., Meilahn E. N., Plantinga P. Prospective study of the determinants of age at menopause. *Am J Epidem.* 1997;145(2):124–133.

Brown A. F., Perez-Stable E., Whitaker E. E., Posner S. F., Alexander M., Gathe J. Ethnic differences in hormone replacement prescribing patterns. *JGIM.* 1999;14:663–669.

Brown J. S., Grady D., Ouslander J. G., Herzog A. R., Varner R. E., Posner S. F. Prevalence of urinary incontinence and associated risk factors in post-menopausal women. Heart & Estrogen/Progestin Replacement Study (HERS) Research Group. *Obste Gyneco.* 1999;94(1):66–70.

Brown K. H., Hammond C. B. Urogenital atrophy. *Obste Gynecol Clin N Am.* 1987;14(1):13–32.

Callens A., Vaillant L., Lecomte P., Berson M., Gall Y., Lorette G. Does hormonal skin aging exist? A study of the influence of different hormone therapy regimens on the skin of postmenopausal women using non-invasive measurement techniques. *Dermatology.* 1996;193(4):289–294.

Clifton-Bligh P. B., Baber R. J., Fulcher G. R., Nery M. L., Moreton T. The effect of isoflavones extracted from red clover (Rimostil) on lipid and bone metabolism. *Menop.* 2001;8(4):259–265.

Cohen L. Depression rates in perimenopausal and premenopausal women: A longitudinal study (Abstract) presented at American Psychiatric Association Meeting. New York, NY; 2004.

Cohen S. M., Rousseau M. E., Carey B. Can acupuncture ease the symptoms of menopause? *Hol Nurs Pract.* 2003;17(6):295–299.

Col N. F., Eckman M. H., Karas R. H., et al. Patient-specific decisions about hormone replacement therapy in postmenopausal women. *JAMA.* 1997;277(14):1140–1147.

Colditz G. A., Hankinson S. E., Hunter D. J., et al. The use of estrogens and progestins and the risk of breast cancer in postmenopausal women. *NEJM.* 1995;332(24):1589–1593.

Collaborative Group on Hormonal Factors in Breast Cancer. Breast cancer and hormone replacement therapy: collaborative reanalysis of data from 51 epidemiological studies of 52,705 women with breast cancer and 108,411 women without breast cancer. *Lancet.* 1997;350(9084):1047–1059.

Cooper A., Spencer C., Whitehead M. I., Ross D., Barnard G. J. R., Collins W. P. Systemic absorption from ProGest cream in postmenopausal women. *Lancet.* 1998;351:1255–1256.

Coutinho E. M., Segal S. J. *Is Menstruation Obsolete?* New York, NY:Oxford University Press; 1999.

Cramer G., Xu H., Harlow B. L. Family history as a predictor of early menopause. *Fert Steril.* 1995;64:740–745.

Cranney A., Guyatt G., Griffith L., et al. Meta-analyses of therapies for post-menopausal osteoporosis. IX: Summary of meta-analyses of therapies for post-menopausal osteoporosis. *Endoc Rev.* 2002;23(4):570–578.

de Bruin J. P., Bovenhuis H., van Noord P. A. H., et al. The role of genetic factors in age at natural menopasue. *Hum Repro.* 2001;16(9):2014–2018.

DeCherney A. H., Nathan L., eds. *Current Obstetric & Gynecologic Diagnosis & Treatment.* New York, NY: McGraw-Hill; 2003.

Decker G. M., Meyers J. Commonly used herbs: Implications for clinical practice. *Clin J Oncol Nurs.* 2001;5(2):pullout insert.

Derman R. J., Dawood M. Y., Stone S. Quality of life during sequential hormone replacement therapy—a placebo-controlled study. *Int J Fert Menop Stud.* 1995;40(2):73–78.

Dog T. L., Powell K. L., Weisman S. M. Critical evaluation of the safety of Cimicifuga racemosa in menopause symptom relief. *Menop.* 2003;10(4):299–313.

Dog T. L. CAM approaches to menopause management: The role for botanicals in menopause. *Menop Manag.* 2004;13(Supp 1):51–53.

Dog T. L. Integrative approaches to women's health: A vision for the future. Paper presented at: Women's Health: An Overview, 2004; Baystate Medical Center, Holyoke, MA.

Edlund C., Dijkema H. E., Hassouna M. M., et al. Sacral nerve stimulation for refractory urge symptoms in elderly patients. *Scandin J Urol Neph.* 2004;38(2):131–135.

Eisenberg D. M., Davis R. B., Ettner S. L., et al. Trends in alternative medicine use in the United States, 1990-1997: results of a follow-up national survey. *JAMA.* 1998;280(18):1569–1575.

Espeland M. A., Stefanick M. L., Kritz-Silverstein D., et al. Effect of post-menopausal hormone therapy on body weight and waist and hip girths. Post-menopausal Estrogen-Progestin Interventions Study Investigators. *J Clin Endoc Metab.* 1997;82(5):1549–1556.

Fairfield K. M., Fletcher R. H. Vitamins for chronic disease prevention in adults: scientific review. *JAMA.* 2002;287(23):3116–3126.

Ferguson D. M., Steidle C. P., Singh G. S., Alexander J. S., Weihmiller M. K., Crosby M. G. Randomized, placebo-controlled, double blind, crossover design trial of the efficacy and safety of Zestra for Women in women with and without female sexual arousal disorder. *J Sex Mar Ther.* 2003;29(Suppl 1):33–44.

Fettes I. Migraine in the menopause. *Neurol.* 1999;53(4 Suppl 1):S29–S33.

Fletcher R. H,. Fairfield K. M. Vitamins for chronic disease prevention in adults: clinical applications. *JAMA.* 2002;287(23):3127–3129.

Freedman R. R., Woodward S., Brown B., Javaid J. I., Pandy G. N. Biochemical and thermoregulatory effects of treatment for menopausal hot flashes. *Menop.* 1995;2:211–218.

Freedman R. R., Woodward S. Behavioral treatment of menopausal hot flashes: Evaluation by ambulatory monitoring. *Am J Obstet Gynecol.* 1992;167:436–439.

Gallagher J. C., Fowler S. E., Detter J. R., Sherman S. S. Combination treatment with estrogen and calcitriol in the prevention of age-related bone loss. *J Clin EndocMetab.* 2001;86(8):3618–3628.

Gallagher J. C., Rapuri P. B., Haynatzki G., Detter J. R. Effect of discontinuation of estrogen, calcitriol, and the combination of both on bone density and bone markers. *J Clin Endoc Metab.* 2002;87(11):4914–4923.

Gambacciani M., Ciaponi M., Cappagli B., et al. Body weight, body fat distribution, and hormonal replacement therapy in early postmenopausal women. *J Clin Endoc Metab.* 1997;82(2):414–417.

Ganz P. A., Desmond K. A., Belin T. R., Meyerowitz B. E., Rowland J. H. Predictors of sexual health in women after a breast cancer diagnosis. *J Clin Oncol.* 1999;17(8):2371–2380.

Ganz P. A., Greendale G. A., Petersen L., Zibecchi L., Kahn B., Belin T. R. Managing menopausal symptoms in breast cancer survivors: results of a randomized controlled trial. *J Nat Canc Insti.* 2000;92(13):1054–1064.

Ganz P. A., Rowland J. H., Desmond K., Meyerowitz B. E., Wyatt G. E. Life after breast cancer: understanding women's health-related quality of life and sexual functioning. *J Clin Oncol.* 1998;16(2):501–514.

Gaudet T. W. CAM approaches to menopause management: Overview of the options. *Menop Manag.* 2004;13(Supp 1):48–50.

Gold E. B., Bromberger J., Crawford S., et al. Factors associated with age at natural menopause in a multiethnic sample of midlife women. *Am J Epi.* 2001;153(9):865–874.

Gold E. B., Sternfeld B., Kelsey J. L., et al. Relation of demographic and lifestyle factors to symptoms in a multi-racial/ethnic population of women 40–55 years of age. *Am J Epi.* 2000;152(5):463–473.

Gorski J. C., Hamman M. A., Wang Z., et al. The effect of St. John's wort on the efficacy of oral contraception. *American Society for Clinical Pharmacology and Therapeutics Annual Meeting.* March 24–27, Atlanta, GA 2002.

Gracia C. R., Sammel M. D., Freeman E. W., Liu L., Hollander L., Nelson D. B. Predictors of decreased libido in women during the late reproductive years. *Menop.* 2004;11:144–150.

Grady D., Brown J. S., Vittinghoff E., et al. Postmenopausal hormones and incontinence: the Heart and Estrogen/Progestin Replacement Study. *Obstet Gynecol.* 2001;97(1):116–120.

Grady D. A 60-year-old woman trying to discontinue hormone replacement therapy. *JAMA.* 2002;287(16):2130–2137.

Greendale G. A., Lee N. P., Arriola E. R. The menopause. *Lancet.* 1999;353(9152):571–580.

Grey M., Berry D. Coping skills training and problem solving in diabetes. *Curr Diab Repor.* 2004;4(2):126–131.

Grimes D. A., Economy K. E. Primary prevention of gynecologic cancers. *Am J Obstet Gynecol.* 1995;172(1 Pt 1):227–235.

Grodstein F., Colditz G. A., Stampfer M. J. Post-menopausal hormone use and tooth loss: a prospective study. *J Am Dent Assoc.* 1996;127(3):370–377.

Grodstein F., Manson J. E., Colditz G. A., Willett W. C., Speizer F. E., Stampfer M J. A prospective, observational study of postmenopausal hormone therapy and primary prevention of cardiovascular disease. *Ann Int Med.* 2000;133(12):933–941.

Grossi S. G. Effect of estrogen supplementation on periodontal disease. *Compend Cont Edu Dent.* 1998;(suppl 22):S30–S36.

Grundy S. M., Cleeman J. I., Merz C. N. B., et al. Implications of Recent Clinical Trials for the National Cholesterol Education Program Adult Treatment Panel III Guidelines. *Circ.* 2004;110(2):227–239.

Guttuso T., Jr., Kurlan R., McDermott M. P., Kieburtz K. Gabapentin's effects on hot flashes in postmenopausal women: a randomized controlled trial. *Obstet Gynecol.* 2003;101(2):337–345.

Hales A. M., Chamberlain C. G., Murphy C. R., McAvoy J. W. Estrogen protects lenses against cataract induced by transforming growth factor-beta (TGF-beta). *J Exper Med.* 1997;185(2):273–280.

Han K. K., Soares J. M., Jr., Haidar M. A., de Lima G. R., Baracat E. C. Benefits of soy isoflavone therapeutic regimen on menopausal symptoms. *Obstet Gynecol.* 2002;99(3):389–394.

Hankinson S. E., Colditz G. A., Manson J. E., et al. A prospective study of oral contraceptive use and risk of breast cancer (Nurses' Health Study, United States). *Canc Causes Control.* 1997;8(1):65–72.

Harvard Medical School. *The Benefits and Risks of Vitamins and Minerals: What You Need to Know.* Boston, MA: Harvad Medical School-Harvard Health Publications; 2003.

Hayes K. M., Alexander I M. Alternative therapies and nurse practitioners: knowledge, professional experience, and personal use. *Hol Nurs Prac.* 2000;14(3):49–58.

Hlatky M. A., Boothroyd D., Vittinghoff E., et al. Quality-of-life and depressive symptoms in postmenopausal women after receiving hormone therapy: results from the Heart and Estrogen/Progestin Replacement Study (HERS) trial. *JAMA.* 2002;287(5):591–597.

Horn-Ross P. L., Canchola A J., West D. W., et al. Patterns of alcohol consumption and breast cancer risk in the California Teachers Study cohort. *Canc Epi Biomark Prevent.* 2004;13(3):405–411.

Hulley S., Grady D., Bush T., et al. Randomized trial of estrogen plus progestin for secondary prevention of coronary heart diseases in postmenopausal women. *JAMA.* 1998;280(7):605–613.

Irvin J. H., Domar A. D., CLark C., Zuttermeister P. C., Freidman R. The effects of relaxation response training on menopausal symptoms. *J Psychos Obstet Gynaecol.* 1996;17:202–207.

Ito T. Y., Trant A. S., Polan M. L. A double-blind placebo-controlled study of ArginMax, a nutritional supplement for enhancement of female sexual function. *J Sex Marit Ther.* 2001;27(5):541–549.

Ivarsson T., Spetz A. C., Hammar M. Physical exercise and vasomotor symptoms in postmenopausal women. *Maturitas.* 1998;29(2):139–146.

Jacobson J. S., Troxel A. B., Evans J., et al. Randomized trial of black cohosh for the treatment of hot flashes among women with a history of breast cancer. *J Clin Oncol.* 2001;19(10):2739–2745.

Johnson J., Canning J., Kaneko T., Pru J. K., Tilly J. L. Germline stem cells and follicular renewal in the postnatal mammalian ovary. *Nature.* 2004;428(6979):145–150.

Kang J. H. Dietary influences on developing Alzheimer's Disease and dementia. *International Conference on Alzheimer's Disease and Related Disorders, Philadelphia, PA, July 21.* 2004.

Karram M. M., Partoll L., Rahe J. Efficacy of nonsurgical therapy for urinary incontinence. *J Repro Med.* 1996;41(4):215–219.

Kellogg-Spadt S. When it comes to botanical prosexual preparations, clinicians and consumers beware! *Women Health Care.* Nov 2003;2(11):15–16.

Klatte E. T., Scharre D. W., Nagaraja H. N., Davis R. A., Beversdorf D. Q. Combination therapy of donepezil and Vitamin E in Alzheimer disease. *Alz Dis Disord.* 2003;17(2):113–116.

Klein B. E., Klein R., Ritter L. L. Is there evidence of an estrogen effect on age-related lens opacities? The Beaver Dam Eye Study. *Arch Ophthal.* 1994;112(1):85–91.

Komesaroff P. A., Black C. V., Cable V., Sudhir K. Effects of wild yam extract on menopausal symptoms, lipids and sex hormones in healthy menopausal women. *Climacteric.* 2001;4(2):144–150.

Kriege M., Brekelmans C. T., Boetes C., et al. Efficacy of MRI and mammography for breast-cancer screening in women with a familial or genetic predisposition. *NEJM.* 2004;351(5):427–437.

Kroenke C. H., Hankinson S. E., Schernhammer E. S., Colditz G. A., Kawachi I., Holmes M. D. Caregiving stress, endogenous sex steroid hormone levels, and breast cancer incidence. *Am J Epi.* 2004;159(11):1019–1027.

Kronenberg F., Fugh-Berman A. Complementary and alternative medicine for menopausal symptoms: a review of randomized, controlled trials. *Ann Int Med.* 2002;137(10):805–813.

Kronenberg F. Hot flashes: Epidemiology and physiology. *Ann NY Acad Sci.* 1990;592:52–86; discussion, 123–133.

Ku Y. L. The value of breast self-examination: meta-analysis of the research literature. *Oncol Nurs For.* 2001;28(5):8150822.

Laan E., van Lunsen R. H. Hormones and sexuality in postmenopausal women: a psychophysiological study. *J Psychosom Obstet Gynecol.* 1997;18(2):126–133.

Laufer L. R., Erlik Y., Meldrum D. R., Judd H. L. Effect of clonidine on hot flashes in postmenopausal women. *Obstet Gynecol.* 1982;60(5):583–586.

Laumann E. O, Paik A., Rosen R. C. Sexual dysfunction in the United States: prevalence and predictors. *JAMA.* 1999;281(6):537–544.

Le Bars P. L., Katz M., Berman N. P., Itil T. M., Freedman A. M., Schatzberg A. F. A Placebo-Controlled, Double-blind, Randomized Trial of an Extract of Ginkgo Biloba for Dementia. *JAMA.* 1997;278(16):1327–1332.

Leonetti H. B., Longo S., Anasti J. N. Transdermal progesterone cream for vasomotor symptoms and postmenopausal bone loss. *Obstet Gynecol.* 1999;94(2):225–228.

Lindsay R., Gallagher J. C., Kleerekoper M., Pickar J. H. Effect of lower doses of conjugated equine estrogens with and without medroxyprogesterone acetate on bone in early postmenopausal women. *JAMA.* 2002;287(20):2668–2676.

Ling F. W., Duff P., eds. *Obstetrics & Gynecology Principles for Principles.* New York, NY: McGraw-Hill; 2002.

Lobo R. A., ed. *Treatment of the Postmenopausal Woman: Basic and Clinical Aspects.* 2nd ed. Philadelphia, PA: Lippincott Williams & Wilkins; 1999.

Loprinzi C. L., Kugler J. W., Sloan J. A., et al. Venlafaxine in management of hot flashes in survivors of breast cancer: a randomised controlled trial. *Lancet.* 2000;356(9247):2059–2063.

Loprinzi C. L., Michalak J. C., Quella S. K., et al. Megestrol acetate for the prevention of hot flashes. *NEJM.* 1994;331(6):347–352.

Loprinzi C. L., Pisansky T. M., Fonseca R., et al. Pilot evaluation of venlafaxine hydrochloride for the therapy of hot flashes in cancer survivors. *J Clin Oncol.* 1998;16(7):2377–2381.

Loprinzi C. L., Sloan J. A., Perez E. A., et al. Phase III evaluation of fluoxetine for treatment of hot flashes. *J Clin Oncol.* 2002;20(6):1578–1583.

Maki P. M., Zonderman A. B., Resnick S. M. Enhanced verbal memory in nondemented elderly women receiving hormone-replacement therapy. *Am J Psy.* 2001;158(2):227–233.

Manson J. E., Hsia J., Johnson K. C., et al. Estrogen plus progestin and the risk of coronary heart disease. *NEJM.* 2003;349(6):523–634.

Margolis K. L., Bonds D. E., Rodabough R. J., et al. Effect of oestrogen plus progestin on the incidence of diabetes in postmenopausal women: results from the Women's Health Initiative Hormone Trial. *Diabetol.* 2004;47:1175–1187.

Mattisson I., Wirfalt E., Wallstrom P., Gullberg B., Olsson H., Berglund G. High fat and alcohol intakes are risk factors of postmenopausal breast cancer: a prospective study from the Malmo diet and cancer cohort. *Int J Canc.* 2004;110(4):589–597.

Mayer-Davis E. J., D'Antonio A., Tudor-Locke C. Lifestyle for Diabetes Prevention. In: Franz MJ, ed. *A Core Curriculum for Diabetes Education: Diabetes in the Life Cycle and Research.* Fifth ed. Chicago, IL: American Association of Diabetes Educators; 2003.

McKinlay S. M. The normal menopause transition: an overview. *Maturitas.* 1996;23(2):137–145.

McLean R. R., Jacques P. F., Selhub J., et al. Homocysteine as a predictive factor for hip fracture in older persons. *NEJM.* 2004;350(20):2042–2049.

McSweeney J. C., Cody M., Crane P. B. Do you know them when you see them? Women's prodromal and acute symptoms of myocardial infarction. *J Card Nurs.* 2001;15(3):26–38.

Bibliography

McSweeney J. C., Cody M., O'sullivan P., Elberson K., Moser D. K., Garvin B. J. Women's early warning symptoms of acute myocardial infarction. *Circ.* 2003;108(21):2619–2623.

McSweeney J. C., Crane P. B. Challenging the rules: women's prodromal and acute symptoms of myocardial infarction. *Res Nurs Health.* 2000;23(2):135–146.

McSweeney J. C. Women's narratives: evolving symptoms of myocardial infarction. *J Women Aging.* 1998;10(2):67-83.

Messina M. Soy, soy phytoestrogens (isoflavones), and breast cancer. *Am J Clin Nutr.* 1999;70(4):574–575.

Morin C. M., Hauri P. J., Espie C. A., Speilman A. J., Buysse D. J., Bootzin R. R. Nonpharmacologic treatment of chronic insomnia: An American Academy of Sleep Medicine review. *Sleep.* 1999;22:1134–1156.

Naessen T., Lindmark B., Larsen H. C. Better postural balance in elderly women receiving estrogens. *Am J Obstet Gynecol.* 1997;177(2):412–416.

Nagamani M., Kelver M. E., Smith E. R. Treatment of menopausal hot flashes with transdermal administration of clonidine. *Am J Obstet Gynecol.* 1987;156(3):561–565.

Nikander E., Kilkkinen A., Metsa-Heikkila M., et al. A randomized placebo-controlled crossover trial with phytoestrogens in treatment of menopause in breast cancer patients. *Obstet Gynecol.* 2003;101(6):1213–1220.

North American Menopause Society. *Menopause Core Curriculum Study Guide.* 2nd ed. Cleveland, OH: The North American Menopause Society; 2002.

North American Menopause Society. Menopause: Definitions and epidemiology. Available at: www.menopause.org. Accessed March 29, 2002.

North American Menopause Society. Treatment of menopause-associated vasomotor symptoms: Position statement of the North American Menopause Society. *Menop.* 2004;11(1):11–33.

Onofrj M., Thomas A., Luciano A. L., et al. Donepezil versus Vitamin E in Alzheimer's disease: Part 2: mild versus moderate-severe Alzheimer's disease. *Clin Neuropharm.* 2002;25(4):207–215.

Palmer J. R., Rosenberg L., Wise L. A., Horton N. J., Adams-Campbell L. L. Onset of natural menopause in African-American women. *Am J Pub Health.* 2003;93(2):299–306.

Pandya K. J., Raubertas R. F., Flynn P. J., et al. Oral clonidine in postmenopausal patients with breast cancer experiencing tamoxifen-induced hot flashes: a University of Rochester Cancer Center Community Clinical Oncology Program study. *Ann Int Med.* 2000;132(10):788–793.

Penotti M., Fabio E., Modena A. B., Rinaldi M., Omodei U., Vigano P. Effect of soy-derived isoflavones on hot flushes, endometrial thickness, and the pulsatility index of the uterine and cerebral arteries. *Fertil Steril.* 2003;79(5):1112–1117.

Pernoll M. L., ed. *Benson and Pernoll's Handbook of Obstetrics and Gynecology.* 10th ed. New York, NY: McGraw-Hill; 2001.

Quella S. K., Loprinzi C. L., Sloan J. A., et al. Long term use of megestrol acetate by cancer survivors for the treatment of hot flashes. *Canc.* 1998;82(9):1784–1788.

Ray N. F., Chan J. K., Thamer M., Melton L. J., 3rd. Medical expenditures for the treatment of osteoporotic fractures in the United States in 1995: report from the National Osteoporosis Foundation. *J Bone Min Res.* 1997;12(1):24–35.

Recker R. R., Davies K. M., Dowd R. M., Heaney R. P. The effect of low-dose continuous estrogen and progesterone therapy with calcium and Vitamin D on bone in elderly women. A randomized, controlled trial. *Ann Int Med.* 1999;130(11):897–904.

Reginster J. Y., Deroisy R., Rovati L. C., et al. Long-term effects of glucosamine sulphate on osteoarthritis progression: a randomised, placebo-controlled clinical trial. *Lancet.* 2001;357(9252):251–256.

Reubinoff B. E., Wurtman J., Rojansky N., et al. Effects of hormone replacement therapy on weight, body composition, fat distribution, and food intake in early postmenopausal women: a prospective study. *Fert Steril.* 1995;64(5):963–968.

Rossouw J. E., Anderson G. L., Prentice R. L., et al. Risks and benefits of estrogen plus progestin in healthy postmenopausal women: principal results from the Women's Health Initiative randomized controlled trial. *JAMA.* 2002;288(3):321–333.

Rousseau M. E. Health care of midlife and aging women. In: Burst HV, ed. *Varney's Midwifery.* 4th ed. Boston, MA: Jones & Bartlett; 2004.

Salpeter S. R., Walsh J. M. E., Greyber E., Ormiston T. M., Salpeter E. E. Mortality associated with hormone replacement therapy in younger and older women. *JGIM.* 2004;19(7):791–804.

Samadi A. R., Lee N. C., Flanders D., Boring J. R., Parris E. B. Samadi A. R., Lee N. C., Flanders D., Boring J. R., Parris E. B. Risk factors for self-reported uterine fibroids: A case-control study. *Am J Pub Health.* 1996;86(858–862).

Santen R. J., Pinkerton J. V., Conaway M., et al. Treatment of urogenital atrophy with low-dose estradiol: preliminary results. *Menop.* 2002;9(3):179–187.

Santoro N., Lasley B., McConnell D., et al. Body size and ethnicity are associated with menstrual cycle alterations in women in the early menopausal transition: The Study of Women's Health across the Nation (SWAN) Daily Hormone Study. *J Clin Endoc Metab.* 2004;89(6):2622–2631.

Sarrel P., Dobay B., Wiita B. Estrogen and estrogen-androgen replacement in postmenopausal women dissatisfied with estrogen-only therapy. Sexual behavior and neuroendocrine responses. *J Repro Med.* 1998;43(10):847–856.

Sarrel P. M. Ovarian hormones and vaginal blood flow: using laser Doppler velocimetry to measure effects in a clinical trial of post-menopausal women. *Int J Impo Res.* 1998;10(Suppl 2):S91–S93, S98–S101.

Sarrel P. M. Sexuality and menopause. *Obstte Gynecol.* 1990;75(4 Suppl):26S–30S, 31S–35S.

Sauerbronn A. V., Fonseca A. M., Bagnoli V. R., Saldiva P. H., Pinotti J. A. The effects of systemic hormonal replacement therapy on the skin of postmenopausal women. *Int J Gynaecol Obste.* 2000;68(1):35–41.

Schaie K. W. The course of adult intellectual development. *Am Psychol.* 1994;49(4):304–313.

Scharf M. B., McDannold M. D., Stover R., Zaretsky N., Berkowitz D. V. Effects of estrogen replacement therapy on rates of cyclic alternating patterns and hot-flush events during sleep in postmenopausal women: a pilot study. *Clin Therap.* 1997;19(2):304–311.

Schull P. D. *Nursing Spectrum Drug Handbook.* Chicago, IL: Nursing Spectrum; 2005.

Scott J. R., Gibbs R. S., Karlan B. Y., Haney A. F., eds. *Danforth's Obstetrics and Gynecology.* Philadelphia, PA: Lippincott Williams & Wilkins; 2003.

Shumaker S. A., Legault C., Rapp S. R., et al. Estrogen plus progestin and the incidence of dementia and mild cognitive impairment in postmenopausal women: the Women's Health Initiative Memory Study: a randomized controlled trial. *JAMA.* 2003;289(20):2651–2662.

Sirls L. T., Foote J. E., Kaufman J. M., et al. Long-term results of the FemSoft urethral insert for the management of female stress urinary incontinence. *Intl Urogyn J.* 2002;13(2):88–95.

Speroff L., Glass R. H., Kase N. G., eds. *Clinical Gynecologic Endocrinology and Infertility.* 6th ed. Philadelphia, PA: Lippincott Williams & Wilkins. 1999.

Stampfer M. J., Hennekens C. H., Manson J. E., Colditz G. A., Rosner B., Willett W. C. Vitamin E consumption and the risk of coronary disease in women. *NEJM.* 1993;328(20):1444–1449.

Staropoli C. A., Flaws J. A., Bush T. L., Moulton A. W. Predictors of menopausal hot flashes. *J Women's Health*. Nov 1998;7(9):1149–1155.

Stearns V., Beebe K. L., Iyengar M., Dube E. Paroxetine controlled release in the treatment of menopausal hot flashes: a randomized controlled trial. *JAMA*. 2003;289(21):2827–2834.

Stoll W. [Phytopharmacon influences atrophic vaginal epithelium-double blind study-Cimicifuga vs. estrogenic substances][German]. *Therapeutikon*. 1987; 1(23–31).

Taylor S. M., Kinney A. M., Kline J. K. Menopausal transition: Predicting time to menopause for women 44 years or older from simple questions on menstrual variability. *Menop*. 2004;11(1):40–48.

The Association of Reproductive Health Professionals. *New Dynamics in Health Care: Hormone Therapy and Menopause Care*. Washington, DC: The Association of Reproductive Health Professionals; July, 2004.

The Eye-Disease Case-Control Study Group. Risk factors for neovascular age-related macular degeneration. *Arch Ophthal*. 1992;110:1701–1708.

Thomas A., Iacono D., Bonanni L., D'Andreamatteo G., Onofrj M. Donepezil, rivastigmine, and Vitamin E in Alzheimer disease: a combined P300 event-related potentials/neuropsychologic evaluation over 6 months. *Clin Neuropharm*. 2001;24(1):31–42.

Thomas D. B., Gao D. L., Ray R. M., et al. Randomized trial of breast self-examination in Shanghai: final results. *J Nat Canc Instit*. 2002;94(19): 1445–1457.

Thys-Jacobs S., Ceccarelli S., Bierman A., Weisman H., Cohen M. A., Alvir J. Calcium supplementation in premenstrual syndrome: a randomized crossover trial. *JGIM*. 1989;4(3):183–189.

Thys-Jacobs S., Starkey P., Bernstein D., Tian J. Calcium carbonate and the premenstrual syndrome: effects on premenstrual and menstrual symptoms. Premenstrual Syndrome Study Group. *Am J Obstet Gynecol*. 1998;179(2):444–452.

Tice J. A., Ettinger B., Ensrud K., Wallace R., Blackwell T., Cummings S. R. Phytoestrogen supplements for the treatment of hot flashes: the Isoflavone Clover Extract (ICE) Study: a randomized controlled trial. *JAMA*. 2003;290(2):207–214.

Unfer V., Casini M. L., Costabile L., Mignosa M., Gerli S., DiRenzo G. C. Endometrial effects of long-term treatment with phytoestrogens: a randomized, double-blind, placebo-controlled study. *Fertil Steril* 2004;82:145–148.

US Department of Health and Human Services. *Clinician's Handbook of Preventive Services*. 2nd ed. Washington, DC: US Government Printing Office; 1998.

Bibliography

US Preventive Service Task Force (USPSTF). *Guide to Preventive Services.* 2nd ed. Rockville, MD: AHRQ Publication No. 00-P046; 2003.

Utian W. H., Shoupe D., Bachmann G., Pinkerton J. V., Pickar J. H. Relief of vasomotor symptoms and vaginal atrophy with lower doses of conjugated equine estrogens and medroxyprogesterone acetate. *Fertil Steril.* 2001;75(6):1065–1079.

van de Weijer P. H., Barentsen R. Isoflavones from red clover (Promensil) significantly reduce menopausal hot flush symptoms compared with placebo. *Maturitas.* 2002;42(3):187–193.

van Meurs J. B. J., Dhonukshe-Rutten R. A. M., Pluijm S. M. F., et al. Homocysteine levels and the risk of osteoporotic fracture. *NEJM.* 2004;350(20):2033–2041.

Varila E., Rantala I., Oikarinen A., et al. The effect of topical oestradiol on skin collagen of postmenopausal women. *Brit J Obstet Gynaecol.* 1995;102(12):985–989.

Vingerling J. R., Dielemans I., Bots M. L., Hofman A., Grobbee D. E., de Jong P. T. Age-related macular degeneration is associated with atherosclerosis. The Rotterdam Study. *Am J Epid.* 1995;142(4):404–409.

Vivekananthan D. P., Penn M. S., Sapp S. K., Hsu A., Topol E. J. Use of antioxidant vitamins for the prevention of cardiovascular disease: Meta-analysis of randomized trials. *Lancet.* 2003;361(9374):2017–2023.

Whitemen M. K., Staropoli C. A., Langenberg P. W., McCarter R. J., Kjerulff K. H., Flaws J. A. Smoking, body mass, and hot flashes in women. *Obste Gynecol.* 2003;101(2):264–272.

Wiklund I. K., Mattsson L. A., Lindgren R., Limoni C.. Effects of a standardized ginseng extract on quality of life and physiological parameters in symptomatic postmenopausal women: a double-blind, placebo-controlled trial. Swedish Alternative Medicine Group. *Int J Clin Pharm Res.* 1999;19(3):89–99.

Wood C. E., Register T. C., Anthony M. S., Kock N. D., Cline J. M. Breast and uterine effects of soy isoflavones and conjugated equine estrogens in postmenopausal female monkeys. *J Clin Endoc Metab.* 2004;89(7):3462–3468.

Woods N. F., Mitchell E. S. Anticipating menopause: observations from the Seattle Midlife Women's Health Study. *Menop.* 1999;6(2):167–173.

Wren B. G., Champion S. M., Willetts K., Manga R. Z., Eden J. A. Transdermal progesterone and its effect on vasomotor symptoms, blood lipid levels, bone metabolic markers, moods, and quality of life for postmenopausal women. *Menop.* 2003;10(1):13–18.

Wyon Y., Lindgren R., Lundberg T., Hammar M. Effects of acupuncture on climacteric vasomotor symptoms, quality of life, and urinary excretion of neuro-peptides among postmenopausal women. *Menop.* 1995;2:3–12.

Youngkin E. Q., Davis M. S. *Women's Health: A Primary Care Clinical Guide.* 3rd ed. Upper Saddle River, NJ: Pearson Prentice Hall; 2004.

Zandi P. P., Carlson M. C., Plassman B. L., et al. Hormone replacement ther-apy and incidence of Alzheimer disease in older women: the Cache County Study. *JAMA.* 2002;288(17):2123–2129.

Bibliography

Index